Health Impact Assessment and policy development

Manchester University Press

Health Impact Assessment and Policy Development

The Republic of Ireland and Northern Ireland

Monica O'Mullane

MANCHESTER UNIVERSITY PRESS

Published by Manchester University Press
Altrincham Street, Manchester M1 7JA
www.manchesteruniversitypress.co.uk

British Library Cataloguing-in-Publication Data
A catalogue record for this book is available from the British Library

Library of Congress Cataloging-in-Publication Data applied for

ISBN 978 0 7190 9193 3 hardback

First published 2015

Typeset by Out of House Publishing
Printed in Great Britain
by CPI Group (UK) Ltd, Croydon CR0 4YY

Contents

Figures

Tables

Foreword

Owen Metcalfe

The public health challenges facing the island include an ageing population, increases in chronic conditions, an obesity epidemic, rising suicide rates, continuing devastation caused by tobacco consumption and excessive alcohol use and an intractable socio-economic gradient attaching to life expectancy and healthy life expectancy. That these challenges cannot be dealt with by the health sector alone is a long standing mantra of those who adopt a social determinants of health perspective. Engagement by other sectors in confronting these challenges can be supported by HIA but adoption of a health lens approach by other sectors is a task that is not without its own challenges. I am delighted with the publication of *Health Impact Assessment and Policy Development: The Republic of Ireland and Northern Ireland* which addresses the situation in Ireland. New public health policies in Ireland, North and South, emphasising a desire to adopt a health in all policies approach and tackle health inequalities are testimony to increasing awareness of the contribution other sectors make to health. However the health lens perspective is not routinely or systematically adopted. It is disappointing that support for HIA and a health in all policies approach is too often characterised as existing by virtue of an individual champion or on a one off basis with respect to a specific initiative or policy. Previous authors have identified numerous barriers to adoption of a health lens approach, including assessment overload, the methodology is too time consuming and burdensome, lack of resources and capacity. These issues and more are explained in a systematic, robust manner in this illuminating volume. When we consider the benefits good health bestows on individuals, neighbourhoods and societies, enabling more to experience the joy of well-being, these barriers must be understood and surmounted. Monica O'Mullane in this volume demonstrates academic rigour, intellectual understanding, huge commitment and a personable approach in furthering our understanding of the role HIA has to play in making this world more equitable and a healthier place in which to be born, grow up, work, play and die.

Owen Metcalfe
Chief Executive
Institute of Public Health in Ireland

Foreword

Maureen Phelan

The publication of this book I feel is long overdue. As a community activist and a community representative on the Ballyfermot Urban project, I feel that this book would be very good reading for anyone involved in the HIA process or indeed anyone involved or learning about the community development process. My involvement in the Ballyfermot (Dublin) HIA Assessment (in 2003 and 2004) was a very interesting and rewarding process. Prior to the HIA there were assumptions made by all stakeholders involved. There were concerns that the city council were not going to listen to the community and their needs would not be met. There was a lot of consultation and the community were happy that all the stakeholders had come together to work on the issues, as traditionally getting the likes of several Dublin City Council departments, several Health board departments, scientists, specialists and community reps, all around one table, working together, had never been done before. The community's needs were listened to and measures were put in place to examine the issues and find out where the true problems lay and what needed to be done to help in these areas. There were some surprising results and because of our partnership with a research group in Italy working on air quality, we discovered things that they had worked on and we had not even considered and vice versa. There was a lot of learning all around. The conclusions and recommendations were not what the majority of the public would have been expecting, but as a community representative I was happy that proper measures had been put in place and the work was very thorough. I was confident in the fact that I could go back to my community and share the findings and report on which measures were going to be initiated to help combat issues that had been highlighted. I feel that the best way forward is for full and honest consultation and an inclusion of all the stakeholders is paramount in any HIA. I hope this book gives others the information on the process and best practice, as if HIAs are properly carried out, the outcomes for all will be generally positive.

Maureen Phelan
Community activist
Ballyfermot, Dublin
Republic of Ireland

Foreword

Susan Doherty

As a local government representative working across the two jurisdictions of Northern Ireland and the Republic of Ireland on the North West Healthy Living, Community Gardens and Allotments Programme funded under the INTERREG IVA, I would like to share some of my experience of HIA and why I believe this book provides a timely contribution to the field. Partners in local councils Strabane; Donegal; Derry; Limavady and Magherafelt, along with the counterparts in the Public Health Agency and Health Service Executive embraced the idea that health is a shared responsibility and provided the opportunity for people to get involved from the outset through shared community garden/allotment site creation to develop healthy lifestyles. In the North West region, the HIA that was conducted was used to provide a baseline of health status within the North West Region so that the health impact of the various training programmes and events could be monitored against this. The HIA offered the opportunity to research, define and compare health issues using various formats such as consultations and focus groups and focused in particular, on the areas of inclusion, disadvantage and poverty, physical and mental health, community engagement and tackling health inequalities. Conclusions from the HIA process indicated that the earlier you involve people in programmes, in this instance gardening programmes, positively impacts on their garden habits, food choice, social skills, nutrition knowledge and cooking skills. Local community gardens/allotments have a proven ability to combat a varied range of public health and liveability issues across the life course. Clearly the HIA is a worthwhile process, although resource intensive and requires a lot of commitment from a variety of partners. However, it provides local and international evidence-based information which can be used to inform and influence decisions such as increasing accessibility and tackling health issues. From my perspective working in local government, this book illustrates the worthiness of HIA as well as the challenges it poses and faces in both jurisdictions in the times ahead. It would be a useful and interesting read for those working in statutory organisations.

Susan Doherty
Programme Officer
North West Community Garden and
Allotments Programme
Strabane District Council
Strabane, County Tyrone
Northern Ireland

Acknowledgements

As with any text or volume, it is not created in a vacuum without the support and encouragement of a wide variety of people. This book is certainly no exception. First and foremost I am indebted to the participants who took part in the research that informs this book. Without such input, honest discussions and genuine interest, I could neither have completed my PhD thesis nor created this volume. My heartfelt thanks to Dr. Aodh Quinlivan for supervising my PhD work. I am thankful to Aodh for supervising with a perfectly balanced mixture of firm guidance and friendly direction. I am most grateful to the following people for passing on information and contacts when I needed it most during the book's writing: Professor Derek Birrell, Brendan Bonner, Denise Cahill, Tony Doherty, Teresa Keating, Jen Martin, Owen Metcalfe, Joanna Purdy, Aodh Quinlivan, Caroline Smith, Karen Smyth and Andy Walker. My sincere thanks to the encouraging voices that have supported my academic passion for Health Impact Assessment, namely, Ms. Karen O'Mullane, Dr. Emmanuelle Schön-Quinlivan, Dr. Marek Majdan, Professor Colin Bradley, Professor Ivan Perry and Professor Fred Powell. My friends and colleagues in Trnava University (Slovakia) and in University College Cork (Republic of Ireland) have always been a massive source of encouragement for which I never take for granted. My thanks to the staff of Manchester University Press for their support of this volume, and for the insightful and helpful comments of the anonymous peer reviewer. On a personal note, I am most grateful for the many blessings of encouragement that I have received, in particular from Dad, Mum and Stephanie, the Kramář family, my many dear friends, and to Peter, for his anchoring support, much needed second opinions, and tender love, especially in the midst of our looming deadlines, due dates, windows of limited free time, et cetera! This book is dedicated with love to Peter and to our lovely little precious Petra Rose.

Abbreviations

AQMAs	Air Quality Management Areas
BBHF	Brandywell and Bogside Health Forum
BCC	Belfast City Council
BHC	Belfast Healthy Cities Partnership
BMTP	Belfast Metropolitan Transport Plan
CARDI	Centre for Ageing Research Development in Ireland
CAWT	Cooperation and Working Together
CDBs	City and County Development Boards
CWC	Community Workers Cooperative
DCC	Dublin City Council
DHSSPS	Department of Health, Social Services and Public Safety (Northern Ireland)
DLDC	Donegal Local Development Company
DoE	Government Department of the Environment, Northern Ireland
DRD	Department of Regional Development, Northern Ireland
DTP	Donegal Travellers Project
EcCoWell	(Ec = Ecology and Economy; Co = Community and Culture; Well = Well-being and Lifelong Learning)
EFHIA	equity-focused health impact assessment
EHSSB	Eastern Health and Social Services Board
EIA	Environmental Impact Assessment
EPA	Environmental Protection Agency
EQIA	Equality Impact Assessment
ERDF	European Regional Development Fund
ERHA	Eastern Regional Health Authority
HEIA	health equity impact assessment
HFA	Health For All
HIA	Health Impact Assessment
HiAP	Health in All Policies

HIIA	Health Inequalities Impact Assessment
HIQA	Health Information and Quality Authority
HPP	healthy public policy
HSC	Health and Social Care (trusts/bodies)
HSCB	Health and Social Care Board
HSE	Health Services Executive
IA	Impact Assessment
IAIA	International Association for Impact Assessment
IFH	*Investing for Health* (Northern Ireland public health strategy)
IIA	Integrated Impact Assessment
IPH	Institute of Public Health in Ireland
LAG	Local Action Group
LCGs	local commissioning groups
LEOs	Local Enterprise Offices
LTACC	Local Traveller Accommodation Consultative Committee
MGPH	Ministerial Group on Public Health
NEPA	National Environmental Policy Act
NHS	National Health Service
NI	Northern Ireland
NIHE	Northern Ireland Housing Executive
NILGA	Northern Ireland Local Government Association
NISRA	Northern Ireland Statistical and Research Agency
OFMDFM	Office of First Minister and Deputy First Minister
PHA	Public Health Agency
RAPID	Revitalising Areas by Planning, Investment and Development
RoI	Republic of Ireland
RPA	Review of Public Administration
RTS	Regional Transportation Strategy
SA	Sustainability Impact Assessment
SEA	Strategic Environmental Assessment
SES	socio-economic status
SHA	Strategic Health Assessment
SHSSB	Southern Health and Social Services Board
SIA	Social Impact Assessment
SWAHB	South Western Area Health Board
TAP	Traveller Accommodation Programme
UNECE	United Nations Economic Commission for Europe
VFM	value for money
WIFH	Western Investing for Health
WHO	World Health Organization
WHO–UNEP	WHO–United Nations Environment Programme

1

Introduction

A multitude of factors influence our health nowadays, ranging from where you live to how much you earn, from the types of health-related behaviours you engage in, to the policies being developed by our public representatives and state administrators. Certainly, experience and research has shown that the limited view, that health care alone influences our health, is outdated and irrelevant in today's multifaceted understanding of health and wellbeing, as a personal and collective asset. The social determinants of health (social, economic, environmental, behavioural, psychological and structural factors) influence health and wellbeing and are predominantly located outside the health care and health policy sector domains (Wilkinson and Marmot, 2003). In many ways, as a result of the information age, societies and communities today are more informed and vocal than ever before in highlighting aspects of development they are satisfied with or not, in a variety of public fora. However, the ivory towers of policy development can still hide the nuances of proposed initiatives, and in recent years the rise of evidence-based policy-making, in all its forms, from the scientific to the participative, has risen in societal importance. One approach and instrument has been developed in order to assess, however imperfectly, policies, programmes and projects for their impact upon population health, namely, Health Impact Assessment (HIA). This approach seeks to inform policy development with scientific and lay knowledge through its methodology and process. The central theme of this book is to establish to what extent, and in what ways, can HIA inform and influence policy development in two geographically close but administratively different jurisdictions on the island of Ireland. The meaningfulness of this book is revealed in the need for societies to be mindful of the information and pathways that inform the development of our public policies, and whether or not the initiatives and processes we engage in (in this instance, HIA) actually do what they advocate to do: inform and influence policy for the better.

HIA, the focus of this book and its use in policy development, recognises that health is influenced by a range of social determinants and so it follows that the development of any aspect of the social, political or physical landscape would also have a multifaceted range of impacts. One only needs to observe the building of a new shopping centre or football stadium to realise the extent of the influences the new development will have on the local and wider community. Mostly the policies and practices that influence health are not confined to the health sector policies and practices. A Health in All Policies (HiAP) approach (and indeed a health-in-everything-we-do mindset) is desperately needed to allow a more integrated development of policy initiatives. HIA seeks to address the arising impacts of policies, programmes and projects from both health and non-health sectors, and although the idea of appraising policies, programmes and projects for health impacts is not new, the systematic and participatory methodology within HIA is novel (Krieger *et al.*, 2003).

HIA is a structured decision support instrument and approach that is used 'to systematically characterize the anticipated health effects, both adverse and beneficial, of societal decisions' (Bhatia and Corburn, 2011: 2410). Its intended use within policy processes is a key feature of the approach and I would advocate, most important, because if it is not used to inform policy development in some form or another, then why involve ourselves in such endeavours? HIA has been formed so that it may ultimately improve our public's health. Within public health, there has been a long-time understanding of the social determinants of health and their connection with mortality and morbidity rates. However, the copious amounts of evidence that has been gathered over the decades, which correlates the way that people live with the way they become ill and die, has not been translated into effective and coordinated action by the policy sectors whose policies, programmes and services have created much of the health inequality and inequity (Wise *et al.*, 2009: 172). Much of the skewed distribution of wealth, and therefore health, favours those in society with the factors conducive to pursuing a long and healthy lifespan. HIA is presented to us as a 'structured, transparent method and process to work with other sectors' to assess the impact of policy proposals on the health of populations (and on the determinants of health) (Wise *et al.*, 2009: 172). It certainly is designed to enable greater intersectoral action and the four HIAs explored in this book will look at whether they were able to achieve this to any significant degree. Another important aspect of HIA is that it seeks to raise the awareness among those making decisions at a programme, service delivery and policy level, that their actions, however far removed they may seem, can impact and indeed undermine health (Winkler *et al.*, 2013). Of course, their actions, when appropriately informed, can equally promote and support health and wellbeing. This explains why HIA is at the heart of much work, research and practice in the development and advancement of the healthier public policy agenda – the promotion of public policy which supports and strengthens the determinants of health. HIA also highlights the common relationships between the various types of impact assessments (for example, environmental, social, regulatory and equality) amongst key partners, so as to strengthen intersectoral partnership working towards the promotion of health and improved public health policy (Bos, 2006). However, as noted by Metcalfe and Higgins (2009), informing the policy process with sufficient evidence of health impacts is not enough, as there needs to be a thorough implementation of all policy measures in order to yield results. The necessary action after the informing of policy processes is a significant 'follow through' requirement.

There has been support for this systematic appraisal of policies, programmes and projects at a global level. The Rio Political Declaration on Social Determinants of Health as endorsed by the World Health Organization (WHO, 2011) is a global commitment that calls for action on the social determinants of health so as to reduce health inequalities and improve health equity. Within this declaration, HIA has been advocated as a vital instrument and approach which can allow for intersectoral work so as to address the social determinants of health. The expected result of such actions would be that policies and practices from a policy and governance perspective could be improved in terms of enhanced healthy equity and a reduction of health inequalities. This global call to action echoes down to the national contexts within which state, regional and local governments, municipalities and service providers can work together to promote health and wellbeing. This ideal can become a reality when making sure that HIA is 'fit for purpose' and pragmatic for all contexts, as will be illustrated in this book's case studies. The European health policy framework and strategy, *Health 2020*, endorses this approach also and identifies HIA as a useful tool in assessing the potential effects of policies (WHO, 2013a).

This book is based on a qualitative longitudinal study, which consisted of fifty-eight interviews. Since the time of data collection during the first phase (2007/8 – phase I) and an updating of background information and of data collection (2013/14 – phase II), a significant economic recession had hit the global economy. The economies of both Northern Ireland (NI; along with mainland UK) and the Republic of Ireland (RoI) did not escape the sharp edges of this downturn. This book presents a unique snapshot of the use and feasibility of HIA in the jurisdictions when the financial pressure and economic situation was healthier than the period from 2008 up to and including 2013 and 2014 – the time of writing this book. Integrating HIA within institutional processes and mainstreaming it as a source of assessment information, which includes the vital voice of people living in the areas subject to policy development procedures, to inform policies, requires a variety of creative and innovative ways to perform this task (O'Mullane, 2013). This certainly holds true in times of economic austerity as much as in times of financial surplus (Kelleher, 1999).

Why this book?

There has been a significant growth in the practice and research of HIA over the past twenty-five years (Harris-Roxas *et al.*, 2012). HIA is supported and promoted by the WHO, European Union, and to some extent, the International Finance Cooperation and Industry Associations (O'Mullane and Guliš, 2014). In recent years numerous HIA books have been produced, illustrating the flourishing field from the perspectives of practitioners, academics and policy-makers (Bekker, 2007; Wismar *et al.*, 2007; Birley, 2011; Kemm, 2012; O'Mullane, 2013; Guliš *et al.*, 2014). The purpose of this book is to explore and present the extent to which HIA has been used to inform local public policy, indirectly or directly, or both, by using illustrative empirical data and experiences of people involved in HIAs. This exploration looks at the influences that are possibly affecting the use of HIAs for policy development. It is one matter to conduct a well planned HIA process and to develop a report with representative and evidence-based arguments, findings and recommendations. It is another issue that these findings and recommendations are translated into policy and are implemented as part of policy measures and initiatives (Haggerty and Melnick, 2013: S7). This is perhaps the biggest challenge for HIA and provides the central theme of this book, with an empirical focus on the jurisdictions of Northern Ireland and the Republic of Ireland. Although HIA has been acknowledged as a worthwhile instrument and approach to inform decision-makers (Wismar *et al.*, 2007; Morgan, 2008), how much it is actually used in policy development across the island of Ireland is subject to scrutiny. Are HIA reports being produced and left to gather dust on the shelves of state authorities, glossy evidence profiles unused in the policy process? What influences the use (and non-use) of HIA evidence?

The answers to these questions lie within this exploratory longitudinal study that considers the influences on the use of HIA evidence, using an original conceptual lens which draws from the political sciences and public health so as to structure the analysis of four HIAs. To date little academic work has been conducted in this area and sparse attention has been paid to the use of HIA evidence in policy formulation across the island of Ireland (Kearns and Pursell, 2007). The European Health Observatory on Health Systems and Policies called for each country to investigate this decision-support instrument and approach, as recommended by the pan-European evaluation on HIA effectiveness. Such investigation is required in order to 'explore the usefulness of the concept and the feasibility of its implementation in a specific national context' (Wismar *et al.*, 2007: 28). Therefore, this book explores the contextual conditions of HIAs and their potential to be used in policies is required and is presented in this volume.

Health Impact Assessment: concepts and definitions

The term and wording of 'Health Impact Assessment' reveals its core emphasis: to assess the foreseeable (when and if possible) impacts of all public policies, projects and programmes upon population health. The concept stresses intersectoral partnership on an array of public policy issues, so that people working in economic, environmental, health and community sectors, for instance, can come together with common goals and work together. The aim is to bring about improved population health, and that health risks, as far as is possible in the usage of health estimations, are mitigated.

Although various definitions and meanings of HIA exist, most agreement in practitioner and academic circles centre on the definition drawn up by the WHO, as formulated by HIA practitioners, in the Gothenburg Consensus Paper in 1999:

> Health Impact Assessment is a combination of procedures, methods and tools by which a policy, programme or project may be judged as to its potential effects on the health of a population, and the distribution of those effects within the population. (WHO European Centre for Health Policy, 1999: 4)

This definition was expanded to include the action-orientation focus of HIA (Birley, 2011), which thereby endorses the core purpose of why we have HIA in the first place (O'Mullane, 2013: 10), with an additional sentence at the conclusion of the abovementioned definition:

> ...HIA identifies appropriate actions to manage those effects. (Quigley *et al.*, 2006: 1)

The Gothenburg Consensus Paper also outlined the values governing HIA, stating that it was important that HIA took into account a number of key values which are married to the reality of any policy environment (WHO European Centre for Health Policy, 1999: 4). This connection of HIA with the reality of policy environments will be examined within the book's four case studies. These values include democracy, equity, sustainable development and an ethical use of evidence. In any HIA endeavour these core values should be prioritised when promoting the maximum health of the population (WHO European Centre for Health Policy, 1999: 4).

Arising from the conceptual roots of Environmental Impact Assessment (EIA), public health and health promotion, and policy analysis, HIA could be considered a panacea for a health evidence-based policy-support instrument and approach that emphasises the impact of all public policies on population health. In terms of policy-making processes HIA aims to influence the content and implementation of devised policies so as to maximise the health benefits and minimise the identified detrimental effects of the proposed policy. It is hoped that all policies which are appraised using the HIA framework are prospective, so as to maximise the extent of influence, although that is not always the case (Kemm, 2006). HIA is described as being policy supportive and can add value to a decision by providing analysis of such positive and negative impacts of a specific policy (Davenport *et al.*, 2006). Increasingly the understanding of how to influence policy-making processes appropriately in order to ensure HIA evidence and knowledge use has become one of the most important ingredients for HIA policy adoption.

Throughout the island of Ireland, HIA is best understood by examining the relevant health strategies that affirm the instrument. The National Health Strategy of the Republic of Ireland (Department of Health and Children, 2001) endorsed the use of HIA, boldly calling for it to be used in policy development. In Northern Ireland, the public health strategy (*Investing for Health*, 2002), a cross-departmental document, recognised HIA as a mechanism to reduce health inequalities and as a means of promoting health and wellbeing. Northern Ireland's regional health strategy (*A Healthier Future*, 2005) also advocates the use of HIA as a policy-support instrument.

In the Republic of Ireland in 2013 the public health framework entitled *Healthy Ireland* was released, and within this document HIA is still endorsed but as part of the development of a Social Impact Assessment (SIA) that incorporates the consideration of health impacts. The government ministry responsible for national health policy is the Department of Health, and the Health Services Executive (HSE) and local authorities are the statutory bodies associated with the government ministry in the RoI (Kearns and Pursell, 2011). In Northern Ireland the government ministry responsible for health policy at the central level is the Department of Health, Social Services and Public Safety (DHSSPS), and the associated bodies include the Health and Social Care Board (HSCB), the Public Health Agency (PHA), Health and Social Care trusts and the advisory local commissioning groups (LCGs) to the HSCB and the local authorities (O'Neill *et al.*, 2012). By June 2014, the public health framework, *Making Life Better*, was released in Northern Ireland. This new strategy, built on the previous *Investing for Health* (2002), outlines the vision for HIA within the future of public health action in the jurisdiction, in a similar sentiment as *Health 2020*, as a 'practical tool used to support HiAP' (DHSSPS, 2014: 102). Established as part of the Northern Ireland Act of 1998, also commonly known as the Good Friday Agreement, the all-island Institute of Public Health in Ireland (IPH) is another statutory body associated with the government departments in both jurisdictions. It is funded by both government departments (health ministries). The Institute was created in line with the vision in the Good Friday Agreement that public health development would progress in a cohesive and collaborative manner across both jurisdictions, and is one of the key agencies in the jurisdictions to lead the way for HIA support and development.

The meaning of health: a self-evident truth?

The social model of health and a holistic understanding of health, based on the wider determinants of health, is what is widely accepted as underpinning HIA globally (WHO European Centre for Health Policy, 1999). However, when partners in a HIA process come from a variety of backgrounds and therefore come to the proverbial table with a variety of conceptualisations of health and wellbeing, then one person's self-evident truth is another's fallacy. This is something explored throughout the HIA cases and discussed in Chapter 6. It is vital that all understandings of health and wellbeing within the HIA process, and generally in all public health endeavours, are discussed in an open and respectful manner, and not dismissed by health professionals and their counterparts, in a quest as the 'lay preachers of the modern world' to impose a unified definition of health and wellbeing, but rather to seek ways of working together from the cross-sections of thought and conceptualisation.

Overview of the four HIA cases: physical environment and housing

The implementation of HIA in both jurisdictions in practice has been mostly at a local level engaging with the health service sector, local authorities, a variety of statutory bodies, community groups, academics and HIA experts. In this book four HIAs will be discussed and explored, two from Northern Ireland and two from the Republic of Ireland. These HIA projects (referred to also as HIA cases and HIAs) dealt primarily with the social determinants of the physical environment (including traffic and transport) and housing, although during the process of the HIAs other key health determinants also came to the fore (for instance, community and social networks, public services and education). These HIAs were also key sources of information for the development of local policies and strategies. Each HIA was conducted at local government level in both jurisdictions, and so for the most part, engaged with the local governance structures. Although there is divergence in the degree of HIA outcome report and process information available, each are looked at in terms of the following: rationale, background, stakeholders (decision-makers; community representatives; health and social care professionals; academic experts), methodology, and the policy process and relevant actors envisaged to use the HIA knowledge. The HIAs were chosen on the basis of their geopolitical locations (two in the Republic of Ireland and two in Northern Ireland; see Table 1.1) in order to reflect the all-island practice of HIA in this study. The following outlines an overview of the four HIAs explored in this study.

A HIA was conducted on local traffic and transport in the Ballyfermot community in Dublin. In this area, traffic problems were cutting through the heart of the suburb and it was an issue identified by the local community. The

Table 1.1 Case studies including the relevant setting for the policy use of HIA knowledge

Title of HIA	*Public policy issue*	*Policy setting*
An HIA of Northern Ireland Housing Executive Proposal to Redevelop Dove Gardens Estate (2005)	Housing	Northern Ireland Housing Executive (NIHE); Derry City Council (Derry City Council)
HIA of Travellers' Accommodation Programme in Donegal, Ireland (2006)		Health Services Executive (HSE); Donegal County Council
HIA of the Draft Air Quality Action Plan for Belfast (2006)	Physical environment (including traffic and transport)	Belfast City Council (BCC)
HIA of Traffic and Transport in Ballyfermot (2004)		HSE; Dublin City Council (DCC)

HIA was deemed an appropriate instrument for examining health impacts and was the first one throughout the island of Ireland in the policy area of traffic and transport. It was then led by the health services and the URBAN II programme primarily, supported by Dublin City Council (DCC; local municipality/authority). URBAN II was the Community Initiative of the European Regional Development Fund (ERDF) for sustainable development in the troubled urban districts of the European Union for the period 2000–66. The second HIA examined was one conducted on the Donegal Traveller Accommodation Programme (TAP), a statutory local government programme in the RoI. This HIA was carried out and led by the Donegal Traveller Project, in conjunction with the HSE and Donegal County Council in 2005. The Traveller community in the county suffer from poor housing conditions, linked with poor health status, when compared with the general population. This is reflective of the situation nationally for this community (Department of Health, 2010). Thirdly, an HIA was carried out on the Draft Air Quality Action Plan that was drawn up by Belfast City Council (BCC), Northern Ireland. The draft plan required a consideration of health consequences of the policy, as identified by the Environmental Health Unit/Department in the council as well as the Belfast Healthy Cities officials. Areas in Belfast were identified as having poor air quality and measures were examined as to how such levels could be reduced. The HIA ensured greater community consultation and recognition of the health impacts of the physical infrastructure, namely the roads network. The fourth and final HIA was an urban regeneration project in Derry/Londonderry,

Northern Ireland. This HIA aimed to involve the decanted residents of a social housing estate in the design of their future housing redevelopment. The HIA was initiated and led by the Northern Ireland Housing Executive (NIHE) in conjunction with the local community health forum (Bogside and Brandywell Health Forum), health services, local residents and the housing association.

All four HIAs resulted in greater community mobilisation of social issues and facilitated improved intersectoral consultation across the institutional boundaries that normally deal with the social and health related issues such as housing, physical environment and community inclusion. The longitudinal study upon which this book is based explored the *extent* of the use of each HIA in policy adoption after the process was completed. The contextual influences were examined which may explain and explore use and non-use, in the aftermath of the HIA process. This book is not solely investigating the use but to what extent HIAs were used, because more often than not, evidence and knowledge that informs the policy process occurs in a variety of direct and indirect ways.

Other initiatives include HIA, which can promote its continued practice. This seems to be the case on the island of Ireland at the moment. For instance, the central role it plays in the WHO Healthy Cities project, established in 1986, illustrates its importance and activity. The goal of the Healthy Cities project was initially to provide a local basis for implementing the WHO strategy Health For All (HFA) and the Ottawa Charter for Health Promotion, and has grown ever since (Barton and Tsourou, 2000; Devlin, 2013). In the Republic of Ireland, Cork, Galway and Waterford are the designated Healthy Cities in phase V (2009–13) and in Northern Ireland, Belfast and Derry/Londonderry are the designated WHO Healthy Cities. The practice of HIA is widespread across the world, with more activity being generated in previously unchartered areas for HIA such as in China, South Korea and parts of South America and Africa. Whilst some countries have institutionalised HIA somewhat at a national policy-making level (or at least, have the experience of doing so), such as in the Netherlands and Canada, most countries' HIA activity is at local government level (Davenport *et al.*, 2006). HIA also belongs within the family of Impact Assessments (IAs) and much work has gone into examining a greater integration of health considerations across the IAs (Fehr *et al.*, 2014).

HIA is well-placed within the literature (Chapter 2) and the health system and local government settings (Chapter 3). The rationale for the longitudinal study conducted for this book is established by the gap in existing research; similar-type research has been conducted elsewhere, including the Netherlands (Putters, 2005; Bekker, 2007) Wales (Elliott and Francis, 2005), Slovenia (Lock *et al.*, 2003), the United Kingdom (Davenport *et al.*, 2006), New Zealand (Morgan, 2008), and across Europe (Wismar *et al.*, 2007). It has not yet been conducted solely in the jurisdictions on the island of Ireland using a conceptual lens drawing from the theories of political science and public health. The range of issues at the foci of the four HIA cases, and their varying geopolitical locations, adds depth of knowledge to this book. The HIAs described and discussed in this book were the 'firsts' in their topic area, that is to say, each one was the first HIA of a particular topic (social housing, TAP, traffic and transport, Draft Air Quality Action Plan) on the island of Ireland.

This exploration of HIA has been structured by drawing from a number of political science and public health theories and schools of thought so as to frame a conceptual lens. This endeavour allows us to look closely at the four HIAs with the same conceptual lens and draw a final conclusion – how and why was the HIA used, or not, and to what extent. Institutionalist (structure-orientation), discourse analysis and impact assessment (values-orientation) and knowledge utilisation theories (policy analysis), form the conceptual lens used to explore each HIA, and then allows an analysis across the four case studies. The perspectives of those who participated in the HIA steering groups (which were made up of local authority decision-makers, statutory health practitioners, community representatives and local agencies) within phase I (2007/8) are examined using the conceptual lens. The second phase of the study (2013/14) explored the longer term impact of the HIAs in terms of policy development and other impacts.

HIAs *should* incorporate available evidence from processes and reports into policy concerns; HIAs *should* influence the policy process. An expectation of the HIA process has established this normative underpinning. This book is positioned to explore whether this is the case or not, and can it be the case in the future? Are we heading in the direction of greater acceptance of all sources of evidence and information for policy development, or is there less consideration of such instruments which seek to penetrate the policy development process at various points of entry? Therefore, a normative understanding underpins this study of HIA.

Wismar *et al.* (2007) conducted a European-wide evaluation of the effectiveness of HIA in policy formulation. This systematic review was long overdue as no methodical appraisal of HIA effectiveness within policy processes had been carried out previously (Wismar *et al.*, 2007). In terms of assessing the implications of HIA as a policy-aiding instrument, this aforementioned research project pinpointed the influence of the institutional and political context upon the effectiveness of HIA as a decision-making instrument. This was taken into account when developing the abovementioned conceptual lens.

Concluding comments

This book presents a unique snapshot of HIA and how it was used, or not, for policy development in two geographically close but administratively different jurisdictions as part of a qualitative longitudinal study, in Northern Ireland

and the Republic of Ireland. Interviews were conducted with people involved in four HIAs in order to explore how the policy-aiding instrument was used to inform local policy development and initiatives, as well as informants and key leaders of public health in both jurisdictions. So as to structure this exploration, a number of key theories frame the conceptual lens, allowing such a scrutiny. Chapter 2 outlines the main literature in the area and presents the conceptual lens used as a way of analysing the four HIAs. The purpose of the lens is to first find out the influences on the use of HIAs for policy development, and second, when used, the extent of HIA knowledge and evidence use for policy development. This is the interesting point of HIA use in policy development; not only was it used, but how much and to what extent? Chapter 3 provides an overview of the tiers of governance and the statutory structures, primarily the local government and the health systems, which HIA must engage with if it will be used for policy development and strategy information. Chapters 4 and 5 illustrate the four HIAs explored for this book, which involved a total of fifty-eight interviews in total (phases I and II) and field trips to each of the four locations. The final chapter, Chapter 6, provides analysis and discussion in terms of the use of the HIAs in policy development as well as providing recommendations, based on this longitudinal study, for the future of HIA in both jurisdictions, based on the findings of the book.

2

Health Impact Assessment

Conceptual roots and public policy

HIA is a multidisciplinary instrument and approach that makes it an appealing process and endeavour for practitioners, researchers and policy-makers to engage with and use in practice. This chapter will look at the various conceptual roots for HIA, all of which contribute to the form it takes today and how it will develop into the future. This chapter will explore aspects of HIA with a view to painting a clear picture of how HIA has come to take the form it has today, and the variety of roots in its origins. In particular, the chapter will explore the HiAP agenda with health inequalities research being a cornerstone to it, and a major part of HIA, Healthy Cities and the impact assessment movement. Also explored will be the growing literature base of policy analysis, which draws from political science, political economy and social science (Kemm and Parry, 2004). The theories from political science in particular, used to build the conceptual lens that examines the four HIAs in this book, will be looked at from the perspective that they allow for analysing HIA as a policy-informing instrument. Policy approaches that are drawn from the field of the political and policy sciences will be described in relation to their usefulness in examining HIA as a source of evidence and knowledge for informing policies, government strategies and service planning. The chapter concludes with the conceptual lens or framework used to examine how and why (and how not and why not) purposively selected HIAs conducted in two jurisdictions on the island of Ireland informed local policies, action plans, future plans for service delivery and so on, in indirect and direct ways (as described in more detail in Chapters 4, 5 and 6). This exploration of the pathways and connections between the HIA process and policies made locally shows one avenue of HIA impact on local policy development. This conceptual lens will form the analysis of four selected HIAs conducted in the Republic of Ireland and Northern Ireland as to their impact on local policy as presented in Chapters 4 and 5.

Background

HIA is an instrument and approach that supports decision-making in a structured and systematic manner (Bhatia and Corburn, 2011). It can support decision-making in policy and planning 'by analysing the potential effects of a planned action on health' (Pursell and Kearns, 2012: 523). This section of the book provides some background to the HIA instrument and approach, in order to describe HIA briefly and, more so, to lay the foundations for the reading of the four HIAs explored in Chapters 4 and 5. Assessing these potential intended or unintended effects is done by drawing on a variety of data sources during the conduct of an HIA, such as various statistical, toxicological and epidemiological data available on the geographical area(s) in question, quantitative and qualitative research data carried out either as part of the HIA or other research endeavours, community profiles, policy analyses and structured literature reviews. As Kearns and Pursell (2011: 92) correctly point out, the primary purpose of HIA is to provide evidence-based recommendations to influence a policy or project so as to 'maximise health gain and minimise negative outcomes and health inequalities'. HIA is founded on the social model of health, which views health as encompassing many facets and factors that impact health and wellbeing, known as the determinants (i.e. the factors that determine) of health, as outlined also in Chapter 1. Figure 2.1 presents an illustration of the determinants of health, also known as the 'rainbow model of health' (Dahlgren and Whitehead, 1991). The model clearly shows how wide the influences or determinants on health and wellbeing are, and how the health care services are indeed, simply one determinant amongst many. This has led to a consensus amongst practitioners, academics and policy-makers that health care and public health endeavours play a smaller role in determining health than once believed (Morgan, 2006; Eriksson and Lindstrom, 2008). This consensus has grown steadily over the years and can be illustrated clearly by the work and priorities led by the WHO, as will be discussed further in the following section in relation to health promotion, healthy public policy (HPP) and HiAP. This understanding that health is influenced predominantly by factors outside the health care system has been expressed in a variety of notable contexts and declarations, including the WHO Constitution (1946); Alma-Ata Declaration (1978); Ottawa Charter (1986); and, more recently, the Commission on Social Determinants of Health final report (2008); the Political Declaration of the United Nations General Assembly High-Level Meeting on the Prevention and Control of Non-communicable Diseases (2011); and the Rio Political Declaration on the Social Determinants of Health (2011) (Baum *et al.*, 2013: 25).

Since Scott-Samuel's seminal editorial in the *British Medical Journal*, 'Health impact assessment: an idea whose time has come' (1996), there has

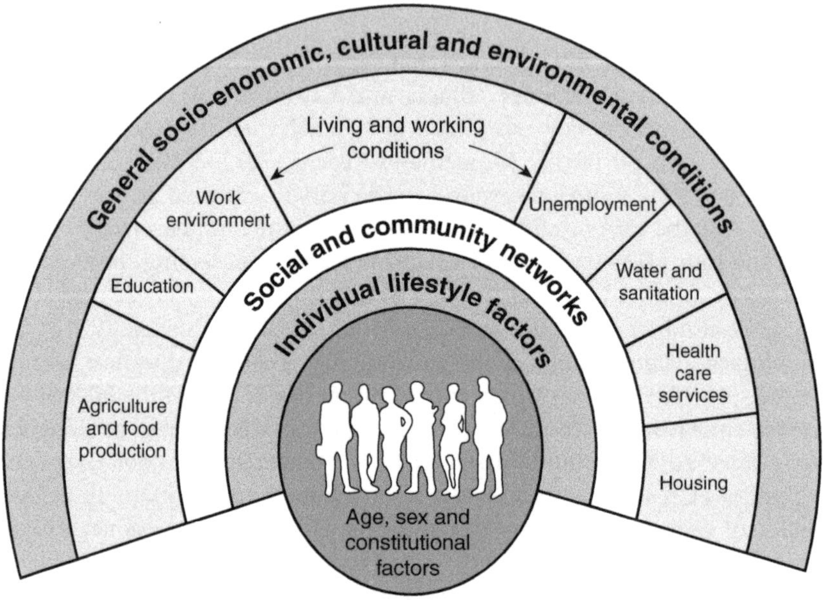

Figure 2.1 The social determinants of health (reproduced with permission from Dahlgren and Whitehead, 1991)

been a growing awareness and increased activity in assessing HIA as a useable instrument and approach to inform local and national policies. Although discussion of HIA had begun in the 1980s and early 1990s, in relation to its consideration within HPP (Milio, 1981) and EIA (Birley, 2003), Scott-Samuel's article initiated the debate of HIA as a feasible instrument for better policy-making. Scott-Samuel (1996) called for HIA to sanction features such as emphasising equitable outcomes, addressing social inequalities, enabling full community participation, and endorsing the use of both qualitative and quantitative evidence. For the most part, the HIAs discussed in this book include such features and illustrate the extent to which, for instance, full community participation can be enhanced.

Putters (2005) states that less focus needs to be spent on defining HIA and more research should be spent on examining the integral relationship between the HIA process and the policy-making arena. The reason for this is simply because, if HIAs are being created but not being used for their intended purpose (to inform policies, programmes, projects and proposals), then the entire process will have been a waste of time, energy and resourcing. It also would generate the feeling that HIAs are not useable or practicable for policy-makers, planners and decision-makers, and so would be ill-considered for use in the future. As Haggerty and Melnick (2013: S7) rightly point out, 'it is one thing to integrate research findings into a report; ensuring that they make their way into policy is perhaps the bigger challenge'. In fact this statement sums up nicely the whole point of this book, to look at whether HIAs are being used to inform policy and their recommendations are being integrated with policy endeavours. The challenge of integrating such HIAs with policy development will be illustrated in Chapters 4 and 5. Much research and effort pre-2005 was spent on defining and understanding HIA, and the post-2005 period was a time for more focused endeavours such as examining HIAs and their relationship with the policy process (O'Mullane, 2013), exploring creative and innovative ways in which HIA, as an approach to implement HiAP, can be integrated with other IA frameworks and with the policy processes (since in most countries, HIAs are not statutorily required) (O'Mullane and Guliš, 2014) and exploring the impact and effectiveness of HIA (Harris-Roxas and Harris, 2013; Guliš *et al.*, 2014). Evaluation will also ensure that the credibility, reliability and appropriateness of HIA processes and methods are useful (Atkinson and Cooke, 2005). Quigley and Taylor (2003) indicate how evaluation and 'tracking' of the policy process, in its acceptance of HIA evidence, is necessary to enable better understanding of the HIA framework.

The stages of HIA are analogous with the stages of other IA frameworks. Diversity in the stages of the HIA process exists; however the majority are based on a six stage model which includes the following steps. The steps are normally carried out sequentially to one another (Metcalfe *et al.*, 2009: 12) although an iterative approach to the process is also a reality (Scott-Samuel *et al.*, 2001):

- Screening
- Scoping
- Appraisal
- Recommendations
- Implementation of recommendations
- Monitoring and evaluation.

There is diversity in how the steps are labelled and in the type of basic model that is adopted by practitioners and professionals. However, generally speaking, these steps outline broadly what an HIA model includes. HIA activities have a number of common features, despite the individual contextual circumstances of implementation (Davenport *et al.*, 2006). Most HIAs use both qualitative and quantitative evidence, they operate within a particular timescale (retrospective; concurrent; prospective), and they range in scope (rapid; intermediate; long-term) (Mindell *et al.*, 2003).

For the purpose of this book, the term decision-maker relates to an individual or group of individuals (deemed the decision-maker) authorised by the state who are involved in making decisions within official state policy processes in some shape or form. This group of individuals (or the individual) is usually in a position of power which is required to make and implement the decision (O'Mullane, 2013). The term 'policy-maker' relates to individuals who develop and inform policy proposals and are often involved in their implementation.

Conceptual roots of HIA and policy history

HIA has grown from a poly-paradigmatic perspective; there is no single distinct conceptual root to HIA, as the influences on its development are varied. The multidisciplinarity of HIA is an important feature of the approach. HIA draws experience and influence from a range of the social, political and environmental sciences, spatial planning, and the public health, epidemiology and health promotion disciplines. Indeed, the multidisciplinary nature of HIA makes it a flexible intersectoral policy-making approach (Bekker *et al.*, 2004; Fabrizio and Paolo, 2011). It is a way of bringing together various partners from a range of disciplines and those working across the policy sectors, for example, transport, education, spatial planning and regional development, and economy. This section of the book will provide an overview of some of the key conceptual roots so as to describe the range of disciplines and endeavours that inform HIA development. This also further contributes to the debates around HIA.

HIA: a key instrument and approach in advancing the HiAP agenda

HIA is very much embedded within public health and has been cited as being born from three distinct areas of activity (environmental health, health equity and the wider determinants of health) (Harris-Roxas and Harris, 2011). It is necessary to approach HIA, theoretically and practically, with a multidisciplinary mindset (O'Mullane, 2013). In terms of the definition of a wider understanding of health, much work has been carried out in advancing the holistic concept of health which today underpins the disciplines of public health and health promotion. There has been much activity at the global policy level from the latter half of the twentieth century onwards. In 1946 the WHO announced its definition of health as being:

> a state of complete physical, mental and social well being and not merely the absence of disease or infirmity. The enjoyment of the highest attainable standard of health is one of the fundamental rights of every human being, without distinction of race, religion, political belief, economic or social conditions. (WHO, 1946: 1)

The definition reflected the circumstances of its birth (after the end of the Second World War) and broadly speaking has stood the test of time despite calls for its redefinition for contemporary times and practices (Saracci, 1997).

The definition, and the concept of health it promotes, made explicit reference to the distinction between illness and health, and how illness alone does not define our understanding of health. The recognition of the social and psychological conditions of health as endowed within the definition have laid foundation to the work of the WHO in advancing the wider determinants agenda for population health worldwide. Health for All by the Year 2000 was a programme of public health reform as declared at the World Health Assembly in 1978 (WHO, 1978). Following the Assembly of 1978, the Health for All Strategy (WHO, 1979) and the Global Strategy for Health for All by the Year 2000 (WHO, 1981) were produced and for the first time at such an international level, stated explicitly that many of the factors affecting population health existed outside the health care sector. This was also highlighted by Marc Lalonde, as Minister of National Health and Welfare in Canada in 1974. The work of Nancy Milio was important in informing the debate around the determinants of health in the late 1970s and early 1980s. Her work and hypotheses informed the concept that we know today as healthy public policy (HPP), which propounds the view that public policy should provide healthier options and support for all policy sectoral areas, which includes health care as one of many. Milio (1981) highlighted the integral role that public policy plays on population health and the importance of assessing policies for their health impacts. In 1986 the WHO released the first charter on health promotion, the Ottawa Charter on Health Promotion (WHO, 1986). Within this Charter, HPP was identified as one of five action areas (which also includes: developing personal skills, strengthening community action, creating supportive environments, reorienting the health services). Since the Ottawa Charter, HIA has slowly but steadily grown as an instrument and approach that can advance the goals of HPP (which involves informing all policy of health considerations), although both approaches can operate independent of one another (Harris *et al.*, 2012). The WHO 1997 Jakarta Declaration on Leading Health Promotion into the 21st Century recommended that policy development should include equity-focused HIA, and almost a decade later the Bangkok Charter on Health Promotion in a Globalised World endorsed HIA as a important tool to aid decision-making (Mindell *et al.*, 2008).

More recently, with the initiation of the WHO-led Healthy Cities movement since 1986 as a local basis for implementing the goals of the WHO Health for All strategy and the Ottawa Charter for Health Promotion (Barton and Tsourou, 2000; Devlin, 2013), HIA has a role to play in advancing the development of this movement in country contexts (Ison, 2009). Additionally, the rise of the HiAP global agenda, as also endorsed by the WHO, particularly since the Adelaide Recommendations on Healthy Public Policy (WHO, 1988), has formed a global movement for integrating a systematic policy health-proofing approach across all government policies (Kickbusch *et al.*,

2008) for which HIA is an ideal instrument and approach. The Healthy Cities movement adopts a holistic view of health, promoting the concept of a healthy city which 'is continually creating and improving those physical and social environments and strengthening those community resources which enable people to mutually support each other in performing all the functions of life and achieving their maximum potential' (Frumkin *et al.*, 2004: 203). Healthy Cities is based on the settings approach in health promotion. The premise of this approach is based on the rationale that it is most effective and sustainable to create healthy supportive environments within the settings of people's daily lives, in the context where the determinants of health interact and affect health and wellbeing. This approach very much mirrors the action areas of the Ottawa Charter (1986) and the earlier Global Strategy for Health for All by the Year 2000 (1981). The work of Charles Landry and his seminal publication *The Creative City* has influenced the focus on creating urban settings that are health promoting, ecologically sustainable and well-planned spaces for people to flourish and grow (Landry, 2008). The work of Peter Kearns and the PASCAL International Exchanges is an example of a platform which brings together strategies and approaches such as Healthy Cities, Green City, Learning City and the Economic Development, to ensure a cohesive movement that fosters quality of health and wellbeing. This approach has been adopted in Cork (Republic of Ireland) which hosted the First International EcCoWell (Ec = Ecology and Economy; Co = Community and Culture; Well = Well-being and Lifelong Learning) Conference in September 2013 as a way of maximising the various strategies that seek to address health inequalities, social inclusion and quality of life (EcCoWell Cork, 2013).

As already mentioned, HIA has been used as an instrument and approach within Healthy Cities as one way of implementing and advancing the goals and priorities of the movement's innovative health actions (Ison, 2009). Indeed, in some Healthy Cities HIA is currently used 'in a more organic way … using a HIA approach within the Health in All Policies process' without following the traditional HIA methodology; taking a flexible HIA approach to project and policy assessment in a context-specific and context-dependent way (respondent from Belfast Healthy Cities). Some Healthy Cities have included HIA within Integrated Impact Assessment (IIA) frameworks (for example, Swansea in Wales, UK) and health-proofing masterplan designs can provide a basis for HIA if one is conducted at a later date (for example, Stoke-on-Trent, UK). HIA, as an instrument and approach, is a very workable way of bringing together relevant partners in assessing the health impacts of projects, programmes and policies. This point is highlighted in this book particularly by the role that Belfast Healthy Cities plays in advancing the HiAP agenda locally by supporting the HIA instrument and approach (Chapter 4).

At the European Union (EU) level, articles of two of its treaties refer to health protection across all public policies. This has emerged as a common health policy theme at the EU level. Article 129 of the Maastricht Treaty (1992) stated that 'health protection shall form a constituent part of the Community's other policies', and Article 152 of the Amsterdam Treaty (1998) called for a 'high level of human health protection (to) be ensured in the definition and implementation of all community policies' (Lock and McKee, 2005: 357). Additionally the European Environment and Health Action Plan (2004 to 2010) (European Commission, 2004) outlined the European Commission's responsibility in environmental and health monitoring, so as to provide Member States with information on how to mitigate negative health impacts of environmental factors and to improve cooperation between stakeholders in the environment and health arenas (Kearns and Pursell, 2011). Accordingly, many policies created within the EU now require a HiAP approach (Council of Europe, 2006; Kearns and Pursell, 2011) for which HIA provides a feasible implementing instrument and methodology. *Health 2020*, the European policy framework and strategy, endorses HIA as a valuable tool in assessing the potential effects of policies, in assessing how policies affect equity and as an approach to strengthen improved coordination of government activities which impact on population health (WHO, 2013a).

HiAP is an approach created to ensure improved governance for health and wellbeing beyond the health care sector and to advocate for health moving up the policy agenda, 'strengthening policy dialogue on health and its determinants, and building accountability for health outcomes' (WHO, 2013a: 14). It is an innovative strategy which focuses on strengthening intersectoral action necessary for HPP (Kickbusch *et al.*, 2008). The approach works to safeguard that all sectors comprehend and act on their responsibility for health, whilst simultaneously acknowledging how health affects all policy sectors. HiAP builds on the work of the WHO Health for All agenda which calls for multidisciplinary action on health; on the concept of HPP as endorsed in the Ottawa Charter; and on the whole government approach enshrined within the Bangkok Charter for Health Promotion in a Globalised World (Wismar *et al.*, 2006). HiAP involves the integration of an awareness of the health impacts of any given policy or programme proposal into the policy development process and ensures the governments address the determinants of health in a systematic way (Kickbusch *et al.*, 2008). In this regard, HIA perfectly fits as an instrument and approach which advances the global agenda for HiAP, from international to local spheres of policy-making (O'Mullane and Guliš, 2014). The HIAs explored in this book illustrate the way in which the HiAP agenda can indeed be implemented at the local level in context-specific ways and dependent on local conditions.

Health inequalities and health equity

As already mentioned, the determinants of health are wide-ranging. They include a variety of intersecting and interacting factors that create and form health and wellbeing (Marmot Review Team, 2010). These influences on health can affect the health and wellbeing of different population groups in different ways, within and across countries and regions, often resulting in health inequalities. Health inequalities are not only to be identified with vulnerable and disadvantaged groups of people, but are evidenced across the entire social gradient, presented as differences in health status across all groups of people (i.e. all grades of socio-economic status (SES); Douglas and Scott-Samuel, 2001). This is an important aspect in understanding inequalities in health as it has been shown, for instance in the seminal Whitehall Study, that differences in health status exist across all groups in society, and these differences affect mortality and morbidity of populations (Marmot *et al.*, 1991). HIA has been cited as an instrument and approach which can concretely address health inequity in its assessment of policies, programmes, projects and proposals (Commission on Social Determinants of Health, 2008), and in tackling health inequalities by raising awareness of inequalities in health, by informing decisions so as to prevent health inequalities in the future and by ensuring more accountable decision-making (Douglas and Scott-Samuel, 2001).

Health inequities occur when systematic differences in health are deemed as avoidable by the taking of action within a society in a country context, or across the wider global society. Health inequities are therefore deemed unjust and unfair. The Commission on Social Determinants of Health (2008) recommended that governments build capacity and knowledge for conducting health equity impact assessment (HEIA) or equity-focused health impact assessment (EFHIA) amongst policy-makers and planners. This recommendation builds on the conclusion of the Acheson report (1998) for the development of a health inequalities impact assessment as a means for examining policies at all tiers of government for foreseen and unforeseen consequences of the policy in producing or exacerbating health inequalities.

Health equity was identified as an integral theme of HIA in the Gothenburg Consensus Paper (WHO European Centre for Health Policy, 1999). Future work and research will be required to make explicit the links between HIA and HEIA, 'and the extent to which they have made a valuable contribution to the range of global activities linked to addressing health inequalities and inequities of policies' (O'Mullane, 2013: 13). HIA is an instrument and approach that addresses health inequalities and seeks to improve health equity in the projects, programmes and policies that it deals with in assessing the foreseen and unforeseen consequences of the proposed action. Although the potential for assessing the impact of public policies on health inequalities and health equity may not yet be fully realised (Parry and Scully, 2003), it remains a useful instrument and approach in considering the differential impacts of public policy (Gorman *et al.*, 2003). As will be observed in Chapters 4 and 5, health inequalities are an underlying theme across the four HIAs explored in this book. It is vital to understand the role that HIA can play in raising awareness of health inequalities and health inequities, and in addressing health inequalities at a local level.

HIA and the family of Impact Assessments

HIA is very much part of a broader family of Impact Assessments (IAs), and draws much of its origin and learning from the experience of EIA. Indeed, environmental health is an identified distinct activity from which HIA was born (Harris-Roxas and Harris, 2011). Various IAs incorporate health considerations to some degree within their frameworks and ethos, including EIA, Strategic Environmental Assessment (SEA), SIA and Sustainability Impact Assessment (SA), in addition to HIA (Fehr *et al.*, 2014). In some country contexts, moves have been made to incorporate health considerations with EIA in order to create Environmental Health Impact Assessments, although the degree to which this happens varies across countries. For instance in India, work has been carried out establishing the degree to which EIA considers health, and the potential for the framework to incorporate such considerations (Cave *et al.*, 2013). Sometimes it is just more practical and feasible to incorporate health considerations within an existing IA, or to amalgamate EIA and HIA, for example, instead of creating entirely new and separated processes. In both the Republic of Ireland and Northern Ireland, as across the EU, EIA is statutorily required according to EIA legalisation and procedural formalities derive from EC Directives, notably Directive 85/337/EEC (as amended in 1997, 2003 and 2009 by Directives 97/11/EC, 2003/35/EC, 2009/31/EC). Unlike EIA, the HIA process is concerned with the means as well as the ends (Banken, 2001). That is to say, the process of the HIA, which involves the networking of the relevant partners across the varying sectoral domains and the raising of health on the agenda of policy-makers, is as important as the outcome HIA report (Mindell *et al.*, 2001). The HIA process is first and foremost, where influencing the policy process is concerned, a political activity and a course of action which requires connection within the political structures (Banken, 2001). From this perspective, HIA is more than the outcome report, as is more the case with other impact assessments.

The EU Directive for Strategic Environmental Assessment was formulated in 2001 (2001/42/EC) and should have been transposed into Member

States' law by July 2004. It requires a consideration of any significant effects on human health and is limited to certain plans, programmes and policies (Birley, 2011). Additionally, the United Nations Economic Commission for Europe (UNECE) protocol on SEA (2003), signed by thirty-five European countries in Kiev, includes explicit references to human health and is based on a broad conceptualisation of health (UNECE, 2003). SEA has the potential to incorporate health considerations to a greater extent, despite limitations such as a separation of planning and health functions in many countries, as well as many spatial planners having little holistic comprehension of the connections between the planning processes and health impacts (Bond *et al.*, 2013).

In Scotland, reviews have been conducted to examine the extent to which health is considered within SEA in an attempt to advance work to ensure that health is adequately considered and incorporated into SEA guidance documents. Additionally, an IIA project was initiated in Scotland which seeks to combine HIA with Equality Impact Assessment (EQIA) and Human Rights Impact Assessment. This IIA was thus named Health Inequalities Impact Assessment (HIIA) and was piloted on seven Scottish government policies and three National Health Service (NHS) Board policies (Douglas *et al.*, 2013). The study concluded that it is easier to bring together IAs with similar foci and emphases (such as HIA and EQIA) rather than those which do not focus specifically on impacts on people, such as SEA. SEAs do not consider differential impacts and therefore do not reflect an equity value (Douglas *et al.*, 2013). This is a useful lesson for Northern Ireland and the Republic of Ireland. Despite parts of IAs including consideration of impacts on health, there currently is no such legal basis for HIA although the environmental assessments must examine the effects on human health. This is a rather narrow focus for population health, on a European basis and within the RoI or NI (or UK) context.

The debate centred on whether an IIA which incorporates all the foci of the various IAs is the best way forward or not, continues. Milner *et al.* (2003) note that an IIA would be more practical from spatial planners and policy-makers' perspectives, however consensus on this issue has not been reached. It is wise to view this issue within the local context in individual states. As suggested by the United Nations (2003: 16), 'local conditions will dictate a specific balance between integration and maintaining a separate profile for health in the overall impact assessment picture'. In Northern Ireland, a Policy Toolkit was developed at the central government level which sought to incorporate the main foci of the impact assessments regularly used (environmental, health, equality). The Policy Toolkit supersedes the previously used IIA. It has been developed and is being led by the Office of First Minister and Deputy First Minister (OFMDFM) in the Northern Assembly.

In the Republic of Ireland a similar toolkit has not been developed although a project conducted in 2013 by the Environmental Protection Agency (EPA) examined the feasibility of legislating for HIA and for also incorporating the instrument and approach into other IAs. The findings of this project were not available at the time of writing, however will make for interesting reading as to the future of further integrating health considerations into IAs and in making a legislative case for HIA in the RoI. In the national framework for action to improve health and wellbeing in the Republic of Ireland, *Healthy Ireland – Framework for Improved Health and Well-being, 2013 to 2025*, HIA is proposed to be included within the recommended SIA (Department of Health, 2013). Although the topic of HIA being a part of another IA or not was not explicitly assessed in the longitudinal study for this book, many interviewees in the research mentioned the practicality of the instrument if it were part of another IA process. This will be further explored in Chapters 4 and 5.

The following section will explore the role of HIA, as an instrument and approach within decision- and policy-making processes, in engaging with communities, specifically with the people who are foreseen to be affected by the project, programme, policy and proposal being assessed by an HIA.

Engaging communities: the role of HIA within the realm of participatory decision-making

Regarding community organisations and broadly speaking, citizen participation in HIA, many practitioners and researchers agree that HIA remains incomplete without both effective and instrumental community participation (NCHPP, 2011). However, the degree to which HIA can enable genuine participation whilst simultaneously improving scientific contribution, is a topic for debate (Parry and Wright, 2003; Kemm, 2005; Elliott and Williams, 2008; Harris-Roxas *et al.*, 2012) as well as in other assessment frameworks (O'Faircheallaigh, 2010; Esteves *et al.*, 2012).

This debate continues to exist between the perspectives of HIA, it being a rational technique (objective) and a social process (subjective) (O'Mullane, 2013). Both approaches existing together may seem contradictory since facilitating public participation and supporting full community engagement in HIA as well as the development of HIA as an instrument that seeks and presents scientific information may prove a difficulty (Parry and Wright, 2003; Kemm and Parry, 2004). As noted in Chapter 1, since one of HIA's key values is democracy, it is vital to consider it in relation to its process and approach. HIA involves the collection of knowledge in order to inform the policy process, and the role of public participation is deep-rooted within both the political nature of the IA framework (Cashmore *et al.*, 2010) and the political nature of the policy system (O'Mullane, 2013).

Birley (2011: 132) reflects that 'HIA is based on an interpretative rather than positivist approach to science'. This does not mean that we disregard and ignore the positivist aspects of HIA since its underlying normative rationality implies positivism. Since we are examining and concerned with HIA as a policy-informing instrument and approach, it belongs more within post-positivism. The tension, perceived or real, between the types of knowledge (objective versus subjective) reflects a historical tension within the policy sciences (Howlett *et al.*, 2009).

Howlett *et al.* (2009) describe the various approaches to policy analysis, including the positivist approach (a deductive and prescriptive one to policy analysis focusing on linking quantifiable policy outcomes with policy determinants), the post-positivist approach (a counter-perspective to positivism, which denies the notion of quantifying outcomes that do not account for social context and the politics of the policy process) and post-structuralist (rejects the presence of objective facts that are separate from subjective observations). It is helpful to be aware of these approaches when reflecting on the HIA process and its relationship to policy development, as they are useful in understanding and analysing policy-making and how its various aspects can co-exist (Knoepfel *et al.*, 2007). It is important for anyone or any group of people seeking to influence the policy process to understand these broad approaches to policy analysis. Regarding the knowledge and information brought together within the context of an HIA, Elliott and Williams (2008: 4) emphasise that the assumption that knowledge gathered by positivist means and knowledge gathered via the lay community are two kinds of knowledge, may lead to an erroneous definition of what is 'legitimate evidence'. There is, however, no reason why both forms of knowledge cannot enhance one another. As Chapters 4 and 5 will demonstrate, lay knowledge and community participation can result in a more comprehensive and in-depth description of the context for the HIA and inform the HIA providing a more holistic picture for the process, thereby leading to an improved process and outcome report, and recommendations for policy.

One question posed by O'Mullane (2013: 30) is 'can these two faces of HIA co-exist without negating one another?' This book responds to this question insofar as demonstrating the important role that lay knowledge plays in the four HIAs examined within this volume, and the way in which such knowledge and community participation lead to greater sustainable outcomes once the HIA process was completed, such as in Chapter 4 where the HIA steering committee for the Traffic and Transport HIA in Dublin (RoI) transformed into a community group overseeing similar actions of urban development, facilitated by the RAPID (Revitalising Areas by Planning, Investment and Development; community-based initiative) coordinator.

The following section will outline HIA's relationship to the policy-oriented approach, and will provide a review of policy approaches relevant to HIA as a policy-informing instrument. The literature of the policy-oriented approach provides a significant framework for the book in exploring how HIA can inform and influence policy development. The role that underlying values and norms play in the policy process, and the relevance of this to HIA, will be discussed. This overview provides a necessary basis for describing the conceptual lens that was used in the first half of the longitudinal study which sought to examine the use of HIA knowledge in local policies in NI and RoI.

The policy-oriented approach and HIA

Before continuing with the chapter, it is important to pause and look at the various understandings of the terms 'policy' and 'politics', and the significance these terms have for HIA. Although much work has been done to date examining the policy process and HIA (Bekker *et al.*, 2004; Putters, 2005; Wismar *et al.*, 2007; Kearns and Pursell, 2011; Kemm *et al.*, 2011; Harris *et al.*, 2012; O'Mullane, 2013; Guliš *et al.*, 2014; Harris *et al.*, 2014), the extent to which HIAs are used to inform policy processes (indirectly and directly) based on empirical evidence has not yet been done within an all-island of Ireland context, and is the subject of this book. A conceptual lens (also referred to as the theoretical framework) that essentially looks at the overarching structures and underlying norms and values (inspired by the work of Bekker, 2007) and that was developed to examine this usage of HIA knowledge for policy development (O'Mullane, 2009a) will be presented in the final section of the chapter. This lens is then used to assess the four HIAs in Chapters 4 and 5 as to how they informed policy development.

As a premise to this section, Powell (2007: 9) reminds us that it is important to decipher the difference between the terms 'policy' and 'politics', as at times in modern social discourse, the terms and underlying concepts are used interchangeably. This can have significant etymological implications. The origin of the term 'policy' comes from ancient Greece (*politeia*) and since those times it was understood as something much more complex than 'politics' (*politiké*). It meant the 'pursuit of civic virtue through good governance' as opposed to the more straightforward meaning of *politiké*, which refers to the art of government. Creating policy, and in fact defining it (considered by Wildavsky (1979) as the indefinable) is such a hugely complex and multifaceted arena that it is unsurprising that it was originally understood by our forefathers as an activity and concept considered the more complex operation of the two terms, despite modern-day confusion between the concepts (politics; policy). It is this complexity that needs due recognition when examining how and why HIA can inform the policy process, in either indirect or direct ways, since HIA must operate in an often irrational and overly complex policy-making environment, as is illustrated by the HIAs explored in Chapters 4 and 5.

The following section of the chapter will outline the various policy approaches relevant in the examination of HIA as a policy-informing instrument and approach, including the perspectives of rationalism and incrementalism, the policy stages approach, New Institutional Theory, knowledge utilisation theories, impact assessment in the policy-making process and the role of values and norms in the policy process. Aspects of these theories, which can help to examine and explain HIA as a policy-informing instrument, will be highlighted and brought together to build the conceptual lens that will help us look at HIA's role in policy development.

Policy approaches and HIA

HIA undeniably operates in a political and policy environment. Within this arena, its proponents seek and attempt to assimilate and integrate its knowledge and evidence within the policy process, so that HIA professionals and practitioners can present policy-makers and decision-makers with a variety of options. These options must explicitly outline their inherent trade-offs, as this information is vital for the policy actors to be mindful of during policy development. Petticrew *et al.* (2004) conducted research with decision-makers regarding their thoughts on how research evidence influences public health policy-making. The participants stated that they seek objective and unbiased evidence as a first and foremost priority. This has important implications for those working with HIA, in that it needs to provide and present evidence in an objective way and to communicate the various trade-offs involved in the presented options (Mindell *et al.*, 2001). This is where the purpose of HIA is somewhat obscured, whether it is primarily an advocacy tool, or a channel for presenting objective knowledge and evidence, or its purpose is to perform both tasks simultaneously (Kemm, 2011). This continues to be a topic of debate for those involved in HIAs and with the policy process, and is yet without a conclusion.

Cashmore *et al.* (2010) rightly point out that IA frameworks are working within or at the periphery of policy processes, and at the very least, are expected to stimulate awareness in policy development of a specific issue. Cashmore *et al.* (2010) identify IA frameworks as policy integration tools, and the extent to which they and their evidence can integrate with the policy process depends on factors such as the actors involved and their range of values and norms, and the barriers and opportunities within the political, institutional and administrative systems. This highlights the importance of understanding the role that HIA can play as a policy-informing instrument and approach. Being aware of the various policy models and approaches which can explain and inform action around influencing the policy process with HIA knowledge can enable a better understanding of how HIA can align itself with such processes. This can lead to greater understanding of the constraining and enabling factors to forming the relationship between HIA and the policy processes.

The topic of HIA and the policy process has been, and continues to be, an area of research and exploration. Bekker *et al.* (2004) investigated the interaction of HIA and decision-making, concluding that by mapping the policy process HIA practitioners can optimise the use of HIA and produce an appropriate HIA. The authors examined rational, incremental and mixed models of decision-making to examine use of HIA evidence by decision-makers. Putters (2005) examined three models of HIA which are connected to relevant policy-making models, namely, that HIA can fit with a rational idea of policy-making, with a rounds (Echternach) model, and with a 'garbage can' model. These models are expected to maximise health interests in policy-making. Research on HIA has also focused on the indirect influences it exerts in informing policy (Elliott and Francis, 2005). Indeed it has been found that effects of policies are oftentimes not realised or experienced by the public for many years after a particular policy action (Scott-Samuel, 2006). Wismar *et al.* (2007) evaluated HIA effectiveness in policy-making by looking at the degrees of effectiveness across various country cases. O'Mullane (2013) examine how the process of integrating HIA with policy can take place, especially given the fact that HIA is not mandatory in most countries and therefore requires creativity and innovation in how it integrates with the policy process. Guliš *et al.* (2014) present an international set of guidelines and approaches which factors in social, environmental and economic health determinants to predict adverse outcomes to populations arising from large-scale policy decisions.

Rationalism and incrementalism

Theorists on the decision-making policy processes have sought to extract the best features from both rational and incremental models, in order to construct a more informed explanatory framework for decision-making.

Howlett *et al.* (2009) notes how the nature of decision-making processes for policy are usually dependent on the policy issue, the actors involved, the institutional and informational contexts and pre-existing decision-making routines and ideas. Such elements are present in some way or another in various decision situations, and the specific nature of each situation will elicit certain approaches to decision-making. There have traditionally been two approaches to decision-making: the rational model (which states that a scientific gathering of information and screening of policy options can be performed) and the incremental model (which states that decision-making has less to do with technical gathering of data and more to do with bargaining and negotiation) (O'Mullane, 2013). Research conducted by Gagnon *et al.* (2007) illustrates the usefulness of taking a subsystem approach to policy-making in their study examining the formation of healthy public policies. In HIA research and practice, practitioners in the field need to be more mindful of the public policy decision-making environment, and as shown by Bekker *et al.* (2004), can adequately inform the process when armed with knowledge of the approaches to decision-making. However, it must still be acknowledged that 'a rational assessment (such as an IA) for an irrational context (policy-making arena) is often difficult' and this inherent tension can at times reduce the impact of the HIA in informing policies and programmes (O'Mullane and Quinlivan, 2012: 186).

The policy stages approach

The policy-oriented approach aims to simplify the complexity of public policy-making into a number of distinctive parts and originates in the work of Lasswell (1959). The stages approach, as it is now known, makes policy more manageable in terms of analysis (Ham and Hill, 1993) although it has not been without criticism (Lindblom and Woodhouse, 1993; Sabatier, 1999).

Lindblom and Woodhouse (1993: 11) remind us that policy-making is a 'complexly inter-active process' and the policy cycle rarely takes the linear form as is theorised. Stages can overlap and it is more useful and practical to view policy-making as an iterative process including these stages than anything inherently rational or linear. For the purpose, however, of examining how HIA can relate to the stages or elements of policy-making, the policy cycle approach provides much needed insight and information (Harris *et al.*, 2014).

There are five stages of the policy cycle. Howlett *et al.* (2009) provides an excellent analysis of these stages, which includes agenda-setting, policy formulation, policy decision-making, policy implementation, and policy evaluation. In relation to the final stage, when combining 'elements of both the positivist and post-positivist perspectives', Howlett *et al.* (2009: 179) can be regarded as a stage of policy learning. The benefit of taking the 'policy learning' approach to evaluation is to broaden the scope for assessing the policy, i.e. its impact on the policy sector, policy actors and in informing future policy directions. Harris *et al.* (2014) suggests that each stage of the policy cycle can be influenced by HIA, whose stages are in turn informing and influencing one another. External to the policy cycle are a number of contextual influencing factors, such as the policy subsystem composed of institutions, ideas and actors. Fundamentally the policy subsystem is made up of policy networks (including interactions inside and outside government between government and social organisations), policy regimes (involves the impact of long-running policy development influenced by actors, institutions and ideas) and policy paradigms (assumptions that may limit action by constraining policy options available). The arena impacts on the policy cycle by constraining or enabling activity, including HIA, depending on the national or local context (Harris *et al.*, 2014; O'Mullane, 2013). Although the policy stages approach was not explicitly used to inform the conceptual lens for examining the four HIAs in this book, the work of Harris *et al.* (2014) enlightened and inspired the form of the conceptual lens.

New Institutional Theory

Along with the development of the policy sciences as a discipline, the study of institutions, as the context framing behaviour and action, began to take momentum. An institution can be defined as 'to include not only formal organisations, such as bureaucracies and markets, but also legal and cultural codes and rules that affect how individuals and groups calculate optimal strategies and courses of action' (Howlett *et al.*, 2009: 44). Prior to the 1960s, institutionalism was an abandoned area of study in political science (Parsons, 1995). However, it is recognised as having an integral role in explaining policy definition and policy-related behaviour, and provides the broadest view on 'the forces that drive the policy process' (Howlett *et al.*, 2009: 43). The acknowledgement of institutional influences on policy development was not present in old institutionalism; this structural influence was considered in a more heuristic light; it 'was a matter of common sense' (Rhodes, 1996: 42). Rhodes (1996) marks the key difference in the traditional 'old' institutionalism and the 'new' institutionalism, as being the emphasis on description and understanding of the former approach, and the more explanatory, methodological and analytical manner of the latter. New Institutionalism focuses on the overarching influences on policy-making in order to explain societal and organisational endeavours underlying policy-making, thus avoiding or overcoming the limitations of individual or group theories (Bekker *et al.*, 2004; Howlett *et al.*, 2009). It proposes an examination of the effects of structures on policy actors, assuming that these structures exert greater influence on human activity than from within individual or group-centred activity (Howlett *et al.*, 2009).

New Institutional Theory (March and Olsen, 1989; 1996; 2005) provides a framework for investigation of the influences upon the use of knowledge for policy development (Weiss, 1980; Rossi *et al.*, 2004; Wismar *et al.*, 2007). As discussed in Chapter 1, the normative dimension in the theory alludes to the norms within institutions that can go some way to explain the behaviour of actors in various institutions and organisations. In an Irish context, McAuliffe and McKenzie (2007) have acknowledged the importance of institutional theory in explaining the trends of health policy-making specifically, by taking account of implicit (such as a changing emphasis of health policy upon a strategic policy vision) and explicit (such as political and organisational leadership) institutional factors. March and Olsen (2005) argue that certain factors can constrain or enable actors to operate within the institutional frameworks, and a comprehension of these factors will facilitate more informed research into the use of knowledge within policy-making, particularly in the use of HIAs for healthier public policy. Previous work has recommended that novel research must be formulated and designed based upon a theoretical framework that will allow for the examination of HIAs from a policy scientific stance. This research has recommended the use of institutional theories (Bekker *et al.*, 2004; Putters, 2005) and theories of policy analysis (Bekker, 2007) for future study into the use of HIAs for policy. These perspectives and recommendations were taken into account in the development of the conceptual lens that was used in the analysis of HIA knowledge and evidence use for policy development for this book, and are relevant in their flexibility of approach for examining such a novel area of research.

Political dimension and institutions

Elliott and Francis (2005) found in their research into the Welsh HIA experience that the influence of the political environment and agenda, and the different interests around the HIA 'table', was considered an important dimension to note when looking at the influences upon HIA knowledge use for policy development. This has also been the conclusion of other HIA research (Davenport *et al.*, 2006; Bekker, 2007; Wismar *et al.*, 2007; O'Mullane, 2013). The New Institutionalist strand of political science theory also contends that the political dimension is an important one to take into consideration, when investigating the influences upon individual and collective behaviour and action (Immergut, 1992; Peters, 1999). Thelen and Steinmo (1992) point out that politics can have as much influence over institutional behaviour (in this case, the use and assimilation of HIAs into policy development processes within decision-making institutions) as institutions can in shaping individual behaviour. The extent to which this dynamic interaction was lived out in the four HIA cases will be explored in Chapters 4 and 5. For this book, politics (the political dimension) refers mainly to institutional and intersectoral politics, unless otherwise identified and stated.

Policy analysis and knowledge utilisation theories

Policy analysis is an area of study that seeks to inform and prescribe solutions and formulae to decision-makers regarding the direction and content of public policies (Weimer and Vining, 1992; 1999). The purpose of policy analysis is to 'deepen, broaden and extend the policy-makers' capacity for judgement – not to provide him with answers' (Milliken, 1959: 167). Political judgement can be understood as using knowledge within a rationalistic model or one of a more pluralistic nature (Steinberger, 1993). Although with different emphases, impact assessment and HIA has a place, conceptually and ontologically, within the policy analytical paradigm (Kemm and Parry, 2004). Stone (2002) has put together a body of work that examines the processes of policy-making and the underlying values and politics which have an impact upon the boundary and scope of policy analysis. This work looks at the extent to which policy analysis can inform, objectively or subjectively (depending on which body or individual is providing the information and the type of evidence being presented), the public policy channels. This research has much relevance to the study of HIA and its relationship with policy development since very often the underlying values and politics at play will influence what evidence is used or not, as is illustrated in the HIAs in Chapters 4 and 5.

Policy analysis, broadly speaking, relates to the analysis of policy options and alternatives (Patton and Sawicki, 1993). By this understanding, the type of knowledge that is fed into the policy process, and the epistemological underpinning of it (Guba and Lincoln, 1989; Rossi *et al.*, 2004), must be taken into consideration (Weiss, 1991; Stone, 2002). In the majority of cases, information does not find its way into policy. Weiss (1977) questioned this rationality of the linkage attributed to this information stream between policy and knowledge, stating that values of the policy actors and researchers, and the reality of 'compromise-making' in policy processes, needs to be acknowledged. Values throughout the policy process are an important consideration, whether implicit or explicit. Weiss (1980) put forward a hypothesis which leans more on the side of incrementalism; that policy develops as a result of 'knowledge creep' and is formulated through a process of incremental decision-making and gradual policy evolution. This was found to be the case in redesigning HIA to integrate health considerations into public policy (Bekker, 2007). The rationalistic approach rejects the political dimension of knowledge utilisation for policy. Knowledge is not often used in a non-partisan, apolitical and objective way. Usually, there exists a politics of use and non-use of knowledge within the policy process; the evidence of certain knowledge put forth may be factually correct but politically inexpedient. This must be taken into account in order to form an accurate picture of knowledge utilisation within the public policy-making process (Chelimsky, 1995).

Weiss (1991) conceptualises this new-found land of knowledge utilisation for policy as adopting a more incrementalist stance towards the domain; a long-term utilisation of knowledge is incorporated into her new hypothesis.

Weiss (1991) categorises models for knowledge utilisation into three groups, as cited in the work of Bekker (2007: 54–5) and O'Mullane (2013: 38) regarding the examination of HIA as an instrument and approach for informing and producing HPP:

1. Knowledge as a provider of facts to fill a knowledge gap.
2. Knowledge as provider of ideas for conceptual policy development.
3. Knowledge as provider of arguments as ammunition in the policy arena.

This categorisation builds on the work of Janowitz (1970) who acknowledged the potential for conceptual utilisation of knowledge over time, labelled as 'enlightenment'. The consideration of politics underlying the use of knowledge and the evaluation of policy rejects the rationalistic approach to evaluation, and recognises the extent of policy learning that can occur in the policy processes. Direct use of knowledge is no longer the only form of utilisation that is recognised, given the political nature of using knowledge in policy (Patton, 1997; Sanderson, 2002).

Rossi *et al.* (2004: 411) have also moved this school of thought onwards with their conceptualisation and the following categorisation of utilisation of knowledge in policy:

1. *Instrumental utilisation*: the documented and specific use of knowledge.
2. *Conceptual utilisation*: the use of knowledge 'to influence thinking about issues in a general way'.
3. *Persuasive utilisation*: the use of knowledge 'to either support or refute political positions – in other words, to defend or attack the status quo'.

A similar typology was also used in the European-wide evaluation of HIA effectiveness for policy-making (Wismar *et al.*, 2007). The meaning of knowledge is a socially constructed concept and term. The underlying meanings and interpretations of the 'knowledge' concept must be made clear at the beginning of policy processes. This point has been emphasised in the work of Bekker (2007), who investigated the policy processes and the way in which HIAs can be redesigned so as to inform policy and aid decisions in the maximum way possible. Policy analysis, as one approach to policy study, and within it the range of knowledge utilisation approaches and frameworks, is one way for practitioners, policy-makers and research to understand and best use the range of knowledge and evidence for policy development.

The policy stages approach is a dominant and sustained approach to policy study (Howlett and Ramesh, 2003). However, it has not escaped criticism (Sabatier and Jenkins-Smith, 1993), as the rationality of the stages-heuristic and the inability of the model to incorporate policy analysis and knowledge utilisation are deemed as hindrances to application of the model to real-world policy study. Theories of the policy stages approach seek to explain ways of change and policy learning in a pragmatic way (Rossi *et al.*, 2004), and in fully understanding how and why HIA can inform policies, it is vital to include the perspectives of knowledge utilisation theories, as has been done in building the conceptual lens that examines the HIAs in Chapters 4 and 5.

Impact Assessment in the policy-making process

Impact Assessment (IA) can be understood 'as a general approach to generating evidence for public policy' since its birth through the National Environmental Policy Act (NEPA) and EIA in the United States (Elliott and Williams, 2008: 3). IAs are generally used in a development project as opposed to the policy context, and from a policy-scientific perspective, they are viewed as rational techniques informing the policy process (Elliott and Williams, 2008). SEA, Sustainability Assessment (Bond *et al.*, 2012), Policy Assessment (Adelle and Weiland, 2012), Policy IA and some forms of IIA are some of the forms of IA that have traditionally focused on the impacts of policy and seek to influence policy. SEA and EIA have paved the way for HIA institutionalisation in many countries, both in terms of the experience of EIA and SEA in particular, and also in terms of incorporating the environmental with health impacts (Dora, 2004).

In addition to the HIA instrument and approach that we know and use in public health and associated endeavours, a policy-focused HIA (referred to sometimes as Policy HIA) (Quigley *et al.*, 2006) is an approach and concept sometimes used to describe activities which examine the impact only of policies on public health (Mahoney, 2009). Joffe (2008) suggested a renaming of what we know as the policy-specific or -focused part of HIA, to be called 'Strategic Health Assessment' (SHA). This is a commendable recommendation, in aligning separately policy-focused HIAs from those performed at project level, since currently the term 'HIA' refers to all types and levels of HIA. However, the SHA term is not in regular use (Mahoney, 2009) and 'the separation of upstream-level and downstream-level HIAs may be a disruptive move for this field of inquiry' (O'Mullane, 2013: 17).

IA is a recognised policy-making tool, acknowledged and used by international and supranational institutions, such as the WHO and EC. It is also a tool that is increasingly integrated and used in the RoI and NI in its various forms. The WHO–United Nations Environment Programme (WHO–UNEP) Health and Environmental Linkages Initiative (HELI) has surmised that IA is an integral 'link' in the policy-making chain, complementing scientific evidence with the politicised processes in which decision-makers operate (WHO and UNEP, 2004). It is deemed a practical tool, which can ensure that both qualitative and quantitative evidence are considered in the decision-making process. This guarantees that more informed policies are developed, as well as strengthening the decision-making process (Corvalan *et al.*, 2000).

IAs, as policy-aiding instruments, are generally categorised under the umbrella of 'rational decision making' or 'rational techniques' (Hertwich and Hammitt, 2000; Kraft and Furlong, 2004). However, these policy-aiding mechanisms can be used successfully, albeit differently, within other decision-making policy models (Bekker *et al.*, 2004; Morgan, 2009). Although a dated text at this stage, Michael Carley's (1980) work provides insight into some pertinent issues surrounding the use of IA frameworks in present-day policy-making (Davenport *et al.*, 2006; International Association for Impact Assessment (IAIA), 2006). While Carley locates impact assessment as being grounded in rational decision-making, he does acknowledge the undeniable pluralistic nature of the policy-making process. No matter how rational or logical policy-makers intend to operate, their institutional setting and context will influence the policy outcome. Instead of bowing to this pluralistic deference, IA techniques must adapt and become institutionalised appropriately into the policy-making arena, whilst accounting for pluralistic decision-making processes.

A major criticism of IAs is that they 'obstruct new development, are overly pessimistic, and generally slow down progress' (Carley, 1980: 138). However, it has been noted by those involved in IA processes (Environmental Protection Agency, 2002; Scott, 2006) that it is a useful tool in bringing scientific evidence to the policy-makers' attention, and in ensuring the local community being affected by development projects, are heard. In policy development the process is far from apolitical, and the information and knowledge as presented in IA reports must adhere to the political nature of the policy-making processes (Deelstra *et al.*, 2003; WHO and UNEP, 2004).

Value judgements

A value is a standard that guides action, attitudes, philosophy, judgement, rationalizations, comparisons, and attempts to influence others (Rokeach, 1973). Recognition of the role which value judgements play in decision-making is essential in comprehending the rationale and formulation of policy decisions (Hertwich and Hammitt, 2000; Bekker *et al.*, 2004; Bekker, 2007). Value judgements relate to the perception of one group of policy-making actors of what a 'good' decision is, which may be the exact opposite perception of another party. Acknowledgement of such value judgements is necessary, as no matter how scientific or rational a policy process may appear to be, it is oftentimes ingrained subconsciously with sets of values, assumptions, beliefs and ideologies of policy analysts and policy-makers.

The trade-offs and value implications that policy options contain must be communicated appropriately and unambiguously to the policy-maker (WHO and UNEP, 2004), in order to ensure the decision-maker is fully informed, both in terms of scientific knowledge, and of the politico-administrative policy context. This has been discussed in previous sections, that the role of HIA and the practitioners leading the assessment, must be to present the information with due cognisance of the inherent trade-offs of the policy options. The following section delves deeper into the role of value judgements and decision-making processes which include IA knowledge, specifically HIA knowledge.

Decision-making models: framing IA techniques

The implementation of IA processes and frameworks has been found to be reliant upon the overall political-administrative context of the decision-making procedures (Morgan, 2008). This has been found to be the case in an examination of SEA practices throughout the EU. Indeed, as much as IA is deemed an appropriate, informative and methodologically-systematic decision-supporting tool, the importance of such tools to inform policy-making remains marginalised to a large extent (Weston, 2002). Most work pertaining to IA is based upon the assumption that by providing decision-makers with predictive and systematic information, the policy-making process overall will be improved (Harris, 2006; Scott, 2006). However, this rational approach, although the logical process all policy-makers probably strive for (Davies, 2000), is not always possible due to a number of constraints. Such limitations, which are the characteristic of real-world decision-making, include cognitive constraints, behavioural biases, and variability of preferences and norms. The distribution of decision-making over actors and time and the concept that the process is one composing of bargaining and negotiation between multiple actors and institutional layers are limitations characteristic of real-world decision-making (Krnv and Thissen, 2000).

One study (Bekker *et al.*, 2004) has examined the use of knowledge from HIA in the decision-making process and how such knowledge use differentiates depending on the decision-making approach. In the rational decision-making model, policy-makers optimise knowledge utilisation and produce policy decisions based upon complete and independent information (Putters, 1996). Alternatively, the incremental decision-making model explains policy-making by conceptualising the process as one where decisions are made gradually, one marginally different decision upon another, and over time and human resources, a decision emerges. The mixed scanning model is presented in this research as being a 'compromise' approach between the rational and incremental schools of thought. In this approach, decision-making is viewed as utilising limited available knowledge and choice, although the sequence of policy-making actions depends upon the overall formulation strategy. Bekker *et al.* (2004) conclude that each decision-making event is policy, time and place specific, and this in turn reflects the decision-making model of the policy in question. By examining the values, beliefs and ideologies of decision-makers, one may elucidate understanding of the reasoning behind non-use of scientific evidence (Cross *et al.*, 2000). In addition, the authors conclude that institutionalism and discourse analysis are other theoretical insights that will further aid understanding of the actor's perspective, and perception, of utilising information in decision-making. These conclusions and findings, and calls for further research, informed the conceptual lens that is used to examine the four HIAs in this book, thus contributing to the overall debate around HIA and policy development furthering the research in this area by building on previous research in the field.

The role of values and norms in the policy process (discourse analysis)

This approach seeks to examine the policy process in relation to language, communication, and systems of beliefs, values and ideologies (Parsons, 1995). As demonstrated in the seminal works of Bachrach and Baratz (1970) and Lukes (1974), policy problems and solutions should be analysed in a way that is at a 'deeper' level than the policy stages or decisional approaches provide in policy process examination. Thus the emergence of 'deep' theories brought forth dimensions and frameworks that enable analysis of policy problems and agendas. Whilst not always empirically apparent, policy problems and agendas may be theoretically investigated through structures of values, beliefs and ideologies (Bekker *et al.*, 2004). This approach provides an alternative analytical lens to the dominant normative and prescriptive policy stages model.

Regarding the relationship between HIA and the policy process, such 'deep level' theories contribute immensely to the analytical lens in examining how and why they are used in the policy processes. These underlying systems of beliefs, values and ideologies can influence the way that HIA knowledge is accepted or not, and used or not.

HIA knowledge for policy development: exploring four HIAs in RoI and NI

Based on the conclusions and discussion of the various approaches to examining policy and knowledge use within policy-making processes as discussed in the previous sections, a conceptual lens was devised in order to assess the use of HIA knowledge for policy development. The purpose of the conceptual lens is twofold: it is to look at the influences on the use of HIA knowledge for policy development, and second, when used, to examine the extent of HIA knowledge and evidence use for policy development. Based on a search of relevant literature, as outlined in the previous sections, the rationale underpinning this study is to assess whether institutionalist structures and underlying values influenced the process of HIA use in policy development, and how this was the case. It was speculated that if knowledge were used from the HIA, then the direct or indirect use of HIAs in policy, and the extent of such usage, needed to be explored. Policy analysis and knowledge utilisation literature informed the type of usage and the extent of usage. In particular, the Rossi *et al.* (2004) typology allows for looking at the indirect and direct use of knowledge.

There was variation in HIA project selection based on the jurisdiction divide. Two HIAs are based in Northern Ireland (Derry/Londonderry and Belfast city), whilst the others are in the Republic of Ireland (Dublin and Donegal). This selection ensured a fair analysis of HIA use across the two jurisdictions, and the variability of the range of HIAs and their locations add depth to the research carried out. In order to explore the use of HIAs and the knowledge they generate for policy development, influences on the use of HIAs were examined. Previous work investigating the relationship between policy processes and HIA use has recommended an examination of the institutional structures and underlying value systems as influences upon HIA use in policy (Kemm, 2001; Bekker *et al.*, 2004; Kemm and Parry, 2004; Putters, 2005; Bekker, 2007; Wismar *et al.*, 2007; Morgan, 2008). Therefore, following on from this rationale, the overarching research question for the study carried out for the book was conceived: how and why do structures and values influence the use of HIAs in policy?

This question asks both a descriptive (how) and analytical (why) question in relation to the factors of influence (structural and value judgements). Therefore, sub- questions are related to the assertion that institutional and value judgements are influences on the use of HIAs for policy. These questions were formulated within the methodological and epistemological approach of case study research design. The following research questions are posed so as to facilitate descriptive and analytical exploration. Chapter 6 seeks to answer these questions, based on the findings from Chapters 4 and 5 after exploring the four HIAs:

- How do institutional structures influence HIA use in policy?
- How do value judgements influence HIA use for policy development?
- Why does the degree of use, both direct and indirect, vary in different contexts?

Figure 2.2 illustrates the conceptual lens for this examination, which draws on the relevant literature as explored earlier in the chapter, and was used as part of a doctoral study (O'Mullane, 2009b). The book is however based on a longitudinal study, which sought to look at how policy development has benefitted in the long-term from the HIAs conducted between 2004 and 2006.

The conceptual lens illustrates the influences on HIA use (institutional; political; underlying belief and value systems). The extent or degree of use was examined instead of whether the HIA were used or not in policy development, so as to allow for a more nuanced exploration, as more often than

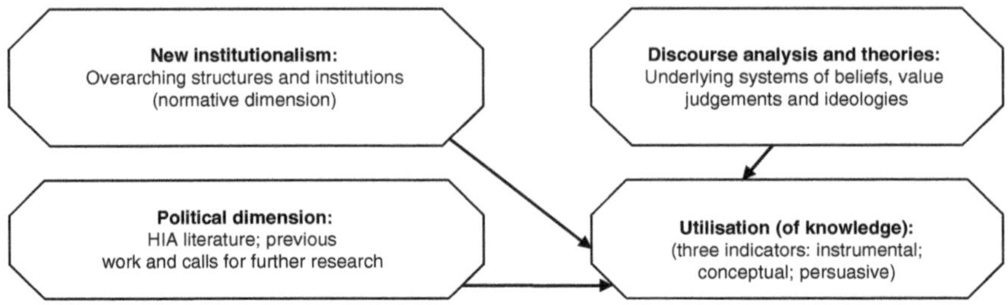

Figure 2.2 Conceptual lens for examining the use of HIA knowledge in local policies in Northern Ireland and the Republic of Ireland (O'Mullane, 2009)

not, it is not possible to assess that knowledge was used or not. Usually it can be used in direct and indirect ways in such complex and multilayered processes of policy development. Each HIA was examined as to the influences on the eventual use of the knowledge and evidence in policy development and also the degree of use in policy was explored. The use of the knowledge gathered from the HIA was assessed in terms of the degree or extent of knowledge utilisation (direct or indirect utilisation). Policy analysis and knowledge utilisation theories informed the way that use of HIA knowledge in policy development was conceptualised. For the purpose of this study, the relationship between the influences and the extent of HIA use is explored in a holistic sense; the influences together are examined and the extent of HIA use is examined, as illustrated in the case studies (Chapters 4 and 5) and in the conclusion chapter of the book (Chapter 6). A longitudinal study enabled an exploration and reflection on the use of HIA knowledge for policy development over a period of time, in this case for the four HIAs, approximately ten years passed since the HIA was conducted and the second and final phase of research carried out.

How the study was conducted

Empirical data needed to be gathered as part of a research study so as to answer and explore the study questions. A case study research strategy was used for this study (Yin, 2003). It was chosen as the appropriate strategy because of the nature of the study: examining four HIA cases which involved both direct observation of events or processes (during the field trips) and interviews with a purposive interview sample involved in the events or processes (in this case, involved in the HIAs). An advantage to the case study approach is its ability and flexibility to incorporate various strands of data sources (Yin, 2003), which has been the situation in this study.

In accordance with Stake's (1995) typology, this research design is a collective case study, as a number of cases were chosen for study to allow for examination of the process and outcome of HIA in each instance. A single case study design was deemed unsuitable for this study as a comparison of patterns and trends in the degree of use of HIAs would provide greater insight to the influence upon HIA utilisation for policy development, and the extent of that utilisation. The HIAs used in this research fit into Hague and Harrop's (2001) classification of cases (representative). They were chosen on the basis of the hypothesised outcome, it being that the HIA was used in some way or another. This selection is subject to criticism as it reduces variation in the cases. However, the literature suggests that the selection of cases along the dependent variable (hypothesised outcome) is feasible, as long as there is some variance in the independent variables and geopolitical context of the cases (George and Bennett, 2004). Therefore, each HIA selected for this research was viewed as a representative case prior to data collection (i.e. typical of the category); each one was completed to the end (outcome reports were concluded in each instance) and all employed internationally endorsed HIA methodology and approaches. The variation in the cases exists in their distinctive geopolitical location, HIA subject matter, stakeholders and partners (actors) and policy environment. From the outset, all were deemed to be similar and representative cases. The extent to which it was the reality of the situation was explored during the data collection phase and thawed out in the analysis phase. It is the *extent* that is being studied and investigated and it is this analysis of the extent of use that provides a wealth of information from the crevices of what is observable from outside.

Qualitative research methods included the semi-structured interviewing technique and participant observation. These methods were deemed appropriate for such HIA research (Thomson *et al.*, 2003). As outlined in O'Mullane (2009b), a case study protocol with a structured topic guide was used during the interviewing phase which was based on the conceptual lens. A purposive sample was selected for those included for semi-structured interviews, which included members of the respective steering groups of the four selected HIAs for the first phase of the study. The analysis included micro (individual actors and their value judgements) and macro (institutional structures and the associated normative and political dimensions) levels of analysis. This is in line with the overarching research question; how and why do the overarching structures and underlying values influence the use of HIAs in policy? This strategy for ensuring a linkage between theory, interviews and analysis is necessary for the robustness of findings and analysis of the research. So as to enable descriptive and explanatory analysis based on the interview data, Ritchie and Lewis' (2003) framework approach was employed. This approach was chosen due to the large volume of transcripts. Text statements from ancillary documents were used to enable analysis of each HIA (for example, policy documents and government white papers) and direct quotations from interviews were used to support the generic themes that arose out of the analysis. Internal validity for analysis was ensured by using the protocol for framework analysis and external validity was guaranteed with inter-coder reliability measures. Two external individuals were involved in the inter-coding activities and more than 90 per cent convergence was reached on the linkage between the direct quotations in transcript data and the codes attributed to them. Interview respondents were asked about their experience in each respective HIA and their opinions on the way institutions worked together.

In the years 2007 and 2008 (phase I of the study), a total of forty-three interviews took place, which was sub-divided into eight exploratory interviews and thirty-five semi-structured interviews with members of the steering committees/groups of the four HIAs. Exploratory interviews were conducted at the beginning of the research when formulating the study questions and when selecting the HIA cases. During each field trip to each of the four HIA locations, additional exploratory interviews that were opportunistic in nature and provided greater detail of the institutional and policy context and narrative that the HIAs are attempting to fertilise. In order to assess the degree of change that had occurred since the original research was conducted and the situation some years later, fifteen interviews took place in 2013 and 2014 (phase II of the study) with a selection of individuals who took part in the original research in phase I as well as exploratory interviews with individuals working within the health system and local government structures. Since approximately five years had passed from the time of original data collection and the re-interviewing phase, many individuals who were part of the HIA steering committees had since moved on to other employment positions. This was a major identified limitation during the re-interviewing phase. As two phases of research took place in two sequential time periods, a qualitative longitudinal study took place to examine the development or progress of increased use of the HIA evidence over a longer period of time. Chapters 4 and 5 describe and discuss the findings from the data collection phases in relation to the conceptual lens, and Chapter 6 presents the analysis of the framework's application. A total of fifty-eight interviews took place. This study and the research that emerged, contributes to the debate around HIA use in policy development by providing empirical data using an originally constructed conceptual lens drawing from the political and public health sciences. This is the first research of its kind to be carried out on the island of Ireland. The use of such a conceptual lens across HIA practice in two geographically close but administratively different jurisdictions makes for interesting reading and a unique and worthy contribution to the HIA debate.

Concluding comments

This chapter presents the conceptual roots for HIA, ranging from the instrument being a key approach to advance the HiAP agenda and tackling health inequalities and inequities, its place within the Healthy Cities movement, to HIA being a member of the family of Impact Assessments. These conceptual roots paint a clearer picture of HIA's form and shape. Clearly, the instrument is influenced by, and equally draws on, a wide range of disciplines and practices, as is also evident when reading the HIAs under exploration in this book (Chapters 4 and 5). HIA as an instrument and approach to enable greater participation of communities in a participative policy process was also discussed, with a recognition of the tension identified between the different types of evidence. The multidisciplinary nature of HIA makes it an ideal intersectoral tool, which is evident from the HIAs examined in Chapters 4 and 5. Policy-oriented theories and their relationship with HIA was explored, specifically with regard to a number of approaches which were then chosen and nested within the conceptual lens used to examine HIA knowledge use in policies in the Republic of Ireland and Northern Ireland. This lens (framework) drew from institutionalist (structure-orientation), discourse analysis and impact assessment (values-orientation) and knowledge utilisation theories (policy analysis) theories. Chapter 6 will describe the way that the conceptual lens has been applied to all four cases and the patterns that arose from comparing the HIAs under the one analytical lens. This study involved using a case study design with qualitative methods in order to examine the structural and value laden influences on HIA use (indirect and direct) in policy.

The following chapter will describe the health care and local government systems in both the Republic of Ireland and Northern Ireland. The purpose for this is to explore the settings or context within which HIA is most likely to engage with a variety of stakeholders, such as a range of statutory bodies, community groups and private agencies. These systems (local government and health) are most likely to adopt or integrate findings of HIAs, as the majority of HIAs conducted in both jurisdictions are at the local level. The four HIAs that will be explored in Chapters 4 and 5 were conducted at the local government level, and understanding the context of the system settings is important in exploring the use of HIA knowledge and evidence.

3

Setting the context for HIA

Health system and local government structures[1]

This chapter outlines the systems of health and of local government that are in place in both jurisdictions since HIA generally engages with such structures. The four HIAs (Chapters 4 and 5) in this book were conducted at a local level and engaged with local government and local health services, which is the more common tier of governance whereby HIAs are conducted (O'Mullane, 2009b; Bacigalupe *et al.*, 2010; Harris and Harris-Roxas, 2010) since the local level of policy-making is considered as having greater flexibility in structure for such policy-informing endeavours (Quinlivan and Schön-Quinlivan, 2009). This makes it more conducive to conducting HIAs (O'Mullane and Quinlivan, 2012). Most of HIA activity is performed at local level, as national policy-making is more contentious, there exists less political will to take on a new mechanism, and national or central policy level HIA has less clarity of function than local level due to the specific targets allocated at the local level (Davenport *et al.*, 2006). This is why it is vital to understand the processes of local policy-making and local governance structures. The similar and diverging characteristics within the systems will be highlighted in this chapter and this analysis will form the context for examining the HIA cases in both jurisdictions. It is within this context that the progress, development and integration of HIA within or on the periphery of the local policy processes in both jurisdictions have influenced the development of HIA practice. This depth of analysis and discussion of the dimensional impact of the governing and health systems from both jurisdictions provides the necessary background for the proceeding chapters on the HIAs that were examined as part of this book's writing. The connection between the development of local government systems and health systems, and their consequential impact on the use of policy-informing instruments such as HIA within the policy process, will be discussed.

Health systems: Republic of Ireland and Northern Ireland

As in all countries and jurisdictions, a mixture of cultural, ideological, economic and political influences combine to structure the contemporary health care system (Quin, 1999). The Republic of Ireland and Northern Ireland are no different in this regard. The influence of its colonial past, post-independence/post-separation political evolution, power balances between the various actors in the health system, and modern-day knowledge and technology in health and disease have amalgamated to weave the system that we have today in both jurisdictions on the island of Ireland (Murray, 2006). This section provides an historical overview of the health care systems in both jurisdictions as well as health policy and the reform agendas. These reform agendas provide the context for the way that HIA will be advanced in both jurisdictions into the future, as will be discussed further later in the book.

Republic of Ireland

Historical overview

The health system of the Republic of Ireland is a unique mix of public and private health care provision. Although the system in place today is closely aligned with the Beveridge model of welfare, the government decided against universal access to care in the 1940s. At the time the dominant Catholic Church believed the expansion of state intervention into matters of the individual and family would be a gross interference into personal and intimate affairs (Fuller, 2004). Also in opposition, the medical profession felt such universality would result in a 'socialisation' of health care, which they believed would be an injustice to the middle and upper classes (Murray, 2006). By inhibiting universality of access to health service these two vocal interest groups, alongside a willing government and a submissive citizenry, ultimately prevented equality of provision (Wren, 2003). The outcome of this was the formulation of the 'two-tier system', described by Barrington (1987: 285) as an 'extraordinary symbiosis of public and private medicine'. As the health system evolved throughout the twentieth century, the inequity of health care access which is implicit in such division between financial means and medical need, is both what is uniquely characteristic of the Irish health system and what is iniquitous of its underlying ethos (Tussing and Wren, 2006).

The Health Act (1970) introduced a restructuring of the Irish health and local government system, since this legislation resulted in powers being transferred from local authorities to the regional health boards. The country was divided into eight regional health boards, in a bid to decentralise health care administration and delivery. The rationale behind the regionalising of the system was to allow local administrative units cater for their local needs, thus taking the health system out of national politics and away from the frenzied media attention and national political machine. It was believed that the result would be improved health policy. Locally elected representatives held places on the governing committees of the regional boards along with ministerial appointments and medical representatives. However, this measure of decentralisation resulted in increased parochialism of health within the regional boundaries and not within the impartial hands of the administration regional boards (McKevitt, 1990).

Health policy and reform

By the end of the 1990s there were deafening calls for reform of the health system from all corners of the health care system, a more vocal society and within the political arena. Reasons for reform included the inequity of access to care and the related debate over the public/private health care provision. The increasing health expenditure that yielded few benefits by way of increased effectiveness and efficiency in the system incentivised the reform agenda. Also the imbalance in the services provided with acute care outweighing resources in the community and in primary care and the increased demands of the populace are further reasons for reform (Quin, 1999).

The National Health Strategy entitled *Quality and Fairness: A Health System for You* was launched in 2001. The health strategy was unique in that it consulted the public, medical profession and other stakeholders during its formulation. Key aims of the reform programme, as highlighted in the 2001 strategy, were to improve patient care health care management, and provide better value for money (VFM) (Department of Health and Children, 2001). In the years following the strategy, changes were introduced into the health system with a view to improving effectiveness, efficiency and patient care. Such changes included the establishment of the Health Information and Quality Authority (HIQA), creation of the HSE (centralised health system which would replace the regional health boards) and a greater policy role for the Department of Health. The Health Act 2004 legislated for these changes, coming into effect on 1 January 2005.

A national framework for action to improve health and wellbeing has been developed also, entitled *Healthy Ireland – Framework for Improved Health and Well-being, 2013 to 2025* (Department of Health, 2013). Goals of the framework include quality of life for all stages of the life-course; reduce health inequalities; health protection; and create a supportive healthy environment (Department of Health, 2013). The plan recommends a whole-of-government and whole-of-society approach to improving health and wellbeing. The framework, and its endorsement of HIA, will be discussed in more detail in the proceeding sections dealing with health promotion and HIA in the state, and its role in providing a vision for the future of public health in the RoI.

Northern Ireland

Historical overview

Similar to mainland UK, Northern Ireland's provision of health and social care became a collectivist mix of 'state organisation and social regulation' from the 1880s onwards until the establishment of the Beveridge universal health system (1948) (Clarke *et al.*, 2001: 32). The British administration's laissez-faire philosophy was replaced by a partnership approach to health and social welfare provision, whereby the state was henceforward the driving force in policy and provision. This policy change accumulated in the establishment of the British welfare regime from 1944 to 1948, in the wake of the Second World War. The newly formed NHS in 1948 was to become the framework within which health and welfare services would be provided and coordinated on behalf of the state. The model of care provision in Northern Ireland was a triadic mix of structures for acute care (hospitals), general practice and public health (Jordan *et al.*, 2006). This structure was in place from 1948 until a change in the organisation of health services occurred in 1974. In that year, Northern Ireland was divided into four health and social services boards (Eastern, Western, Southern and Northern). A defining feature of Northern Ireland's health system is the integration of health and social services in the policy formulation, implementation and provision stages of health care (Jordan *et al.*, 2006). These four boards had the responsibility for provision of services within their assigned boundaries, while the DHSSPS is the leading central government ministry in Northern Ireland to lead the direction of regional health policy and practice.

Health policy and reform

There has been an ongoing reform agenda of the public administration structures and priorities of work in Northern Ireland since devolution in 1999. This process and programme of reform is entitled the Review of Public Administration (RPA). The RPA was conceived in order to ensure that administrative structures were best suited to the needs of the population following the new political context created by the Belfast/Good Friday Agreement (1998) (O'Neill *et al.*, 2012). Local government ministers pledged 'to lead the most effective and accountable form of government in Northern Ireland' (Northern Ireland Executive, 2002: 6). The RPA started in 2002 and concluded with recommendations as part of the strategy document *Better Government for Northern Ireland* (Northern Ireland Office, 2006). Many changes that have been agreed as a result of the RPA are planned to be put into place by April 2015. The reforms relate to local government, educational restructuring, health and social services restructuring and quangos (quasi-autonomous non-governmental organisations) (Knox, 2008). The most pertinent reasons for the health and social services reform were the need to improve the efficiency of resource use and the responsiveness of the care services. The case for efficiency of resource use is pinpointed to public expenditure in Northern Ireland which, for the period 2012/13, was 24 per cent higher per person than the average figure across the UK (Webb, 2014), whilst the revenue raised in Northern Ireland is the smallest of all UK regions. All public sector entities, including the local government and educational authorities, have undergone and continue to experience radical change in their organisational make-up (Jordan *et al.*, 2006). Over time the system became disjointed because of the number of organisations involved in administering care and the centralisation and amalgamation of bodies is hoped to reduce this fragmentation. Such centralisation occurred in the RoI with the establishment of the HSE for the same reason. As a result of the RPA process, the Health and Social Care (Reform) Act (Northern Ireland) 2009 was created. There are currently eighteen bodies administering and delivering care in Northern Ireland. The legislation aimed to ensure that the health system would be more accountable and centred on patient needs. The DHSSPS continues as the strategic controlling authority, whilst the HSCB and the PHA were established under the act and are responsible for commissioning care and five Health and Social Care (trusts/bodies) (HSC) to provide the care (O'Neill *et al.*, 2012). The HSCB is supported by the advisory function of five LCGs.

During the lifetime of the RPA major policy statements were launched to signify the commitment to change and system reform in Northern Ireland. The key areas of acute hospital care (*Developing Better Services*), quality of care (*Best Practice, Best Care*) and public health (*Investing for Health*) have been targeted for action in the programme for change in Northern Ireland (Jordan *et al.*, 2006). In line with the modernisation programme in the health system, a regional strategy, *A Healthier Future*, was published in 2005. This policy document outlines a twenty-year framework for the development of a health and social care service in Northern Ireland (DHSSPS, 2005). During the formulation of the document, extensive consultation was carried out with the general public to ensure that the long-term strategy was tailored to the needs of the service users. There is strong emphasis on coordinating the implementation of the strategy over the next twenty years in addition to public health initiatives, the improvement of multidisciplinary team-working, quality of care, and maintaining care in the community (tertiary care), rather than in acute hospitals. System modernisation in the health and social care services must take place in conjunction with the reform agenda across the UK (Jordan *et al.*, 2006). The strategy published in 2005 is aimed to facilitate reform within the health and social care systems, as well as ensure adequate daily-running of the system takes place on the ground.

Building on the work of *Investing for Health*, an updated public health framework was developed and released by June 2014, entitled *Making Life Better*. Although the framework is not as emphatic in its wording as its predecessor in supporting and committing to HIA, it does endorse the instrument and approach as a practical means of advancing the HiAP agenda.

Although HIA is not visibly on the agenda of the DHSSPS in NI, it may gain greater traction within the newly structured PHA as it is a relatively new agency (established in 2009), as outlined by a respondent interviewed from Belfast Healthy Cities in 2014:

> HIA was part of *Investing for Health*, and the Department of Health (DHSSPS) co-funds the Institute of Public Health. The question is, where is the remit for HIA? Whose responsibility is it to push HIA … In NI, the PHA is a relatively new organisation, it may well come on the agenda now.

The lack of specification of HIA as an area of work for departments, agencies and people working in these organisations is a major barrier to the development of the instrument and approach, as it can only become lost if it is not part of work duties or has a legislative basis.

Local government in the Republic of Ireland and Northern Ireland

This section will provide an account of the system of local government in the Republic of Ireland and Northern Ireland. It is important, within the context of this book and in exploring the four HIAs chosen for study, to have a clear understanding of the policy-making structures and processes in place at local level.

Republic of Ireland

The current system of local government

The following section will illustrate the structure of local government today, in terms of form (composition), functions, financial arrangement, and the reform and modernisation agenda.

Form

The current structure of local government in the Republic is made up of three tiers. The eight regional tiers were introduced to monitor the activities of projects at local level throughout the country. The county level authorities include the twenty-nine county councils and five city councils (thirty-four in total) and are deemed the primary units of local government. At sub-county level, there are seventy-five town councils and five borough councils, which carry out functions for urban areas in particular. The Local Government Reform Act 2014 introduced a structural change that replaced the town and borough councils with a new system of municipal districts. The Local Government (Dublin) Act (1993) legislated for the creation of the only county councils to be instituted since the foundation of the state; Dún Laoghaire-Rathdown, Fingal and South Dublin. The Local Government Reform Act 2014 legislates for reducing the number of local authorities from 114 to 31, completely abolishing the town councils and amalgamating the councils in Limerick, Waterford and Tipperary.

Function

Functions that local authorities undertake can be broadly categorised under the following eight groups (Weeks and Quinlivan, 2009: 11):

- Housing and building
- Road transportation and safety
- Water supply and sewerage
- Development incentives and control
- Environmental protection
- Recreation and amenities
- Agriculture, education, health and welfare
- Miscellaneous.

With regard to local government functions, the Republic of Ireland rates quite poorly in comparison with international countries despite the abovementioned list (Weeks and Quinlivan, 2009: 11). The functions of local government have been continuously eroded over the past number of decades, whereby health functions were transferred to Regional Health Boards (under the Health Act (1970)). The only educational function the local authorities had is an agency one, in the processing of third level student grants. Now this function has been centralised into a system called SUSI. Daeman and Schaap (2000) have concluded that the powers and functions of local government in the Republic of Ireland are narrow compared to other jurisdictions, most particularly in the areas of health, education and welfare. Reasons for the limited functions, and an ever decreasing of these functions as outlined by the Local Government Reform Act 2014, at local level can be understood in the context of central government's tendency to withdraw functions as opposed to supporting local authorities to retain their responsibilities.

Finance

Local government in the Republic is funded through a number of routes, including commercial rates, charges for goods and services, and transfers from central government via the Local Government Fund. Based on 2004 annual figures, charges for goods and services were the most significant source of funding (31 per cent), while funding from central government (23 per cent), general purposes grant (21 per cent) come next in line of significance. Commercial rates remain an important source of revenue for local authorities, providing a quarter of funding (Indecon International Consultants, 2005).

Reform

Contemporary debate on local government in Ireland centres on reform and the extent of it in reality. Comparatively the Republic of Ireland has fewer local government functions than many European partners. This anomaly has been somewhat addressed through measures of reform. Until the decimation of the local functions from the 1970s onwards, the system was adjusting well to the management system with a few amendments to it in favour of councillors (City and County (Amendment) Management Act (1955)). Following the decrease of local authority finances during the 1980s, a decade already in the midst of national economic recession, the 1990s was one characterised by a reform agenda. *Better Local Government (BLG) – A Programme for Change* (1996) is recognised as a seminal policy document, recommending key areas of reform (Department of the Environment, 1996). It set the scene for the reform elements of the Local Government Act (2001). Amongst some of the central aims of this legislation, the most pertinent related to a modernisation of local government law, enhancement of the role of the elected members, support of local interest in policy-making and support the programme of renewal. The key outcomes of the act were the annual representational payment for elected members and the abolishment of the dual mandate. Constitutional recognition of local government in Bunreacht na hÉireann (Republic of Ireland Constitution) which resulted in an amendment to the legal document in 1999 (article 28A) was an important step to ensure that tier of government was acknowledged in the country's basic law.

In relation to local government system reform, the Local Government Reform Act 2014 legislates for the proposals set out in the local government programme entitled *Action Programme for Effective Local Government – Putting People First* released in October 2012 (Department of the Environment, Community and Local Government, 2013). Quinlivan (2013c) notes that 'these proposals by Minister Phil Hogan are a grave concern for those of us who believe in local democracy and local self-government' as the biggest change proposed is to reduce the number of local authorities in the Republic of Ireland by 73 per cent, decreasing from 114 to 31. The complete abolition of all town councils and amalgamations in Limerick, Waterford and Tipperary will enable this reduction to become a reality (Quinlivan, 2013b). *Putting People First*, upon which the Act is based, includes very little reference to local democracy, which is the primary value governing HIA (WHO European Centre for Health Policy, 1999). What is included in relation to democracy specifically is a summary of Part 5 (Chapter 11), where it is mentioned in the last point and 'in the vaguest of terms with a commitment to explore possible participative democracy methods to complement local representative democracy' (Quinlivan, 2013a). Locally elected councillors will lose planning powers they hold under section 140 of the Local Government 2001 Act. Section 157 of the Finance (Local Property Tax) Act 2012 states that a local property tax will be collected from Irish households, however it will be sent to the Central Exchequer as opposed to remaining within the local government financial system. According to the OECD report on Ireland (*Ireland – Towards an Integrated Public Service*; OECD, 2008), a significant reform of the local government financing system is urgently required, proposing more locally based sources of funding. What all of this means is that powers of local authorities will be reduced in the Republic of Ireland. This will impact negatively on how the HIA instrument and approach is to involve this key stakeholder. In the two HIA cases discussed in Chapter 4, the local authority was a key stakeholder and partner in the HIA, since the policies being assessed by the instrument originated from the local authority. The financial and workload pressure on local government, the reduction of powers within the authorities and the outright abolition of local authorities will mean that engaging with such entities will become more challenging.

The Local Government Reform Act also made changes to community development in the context of local government, by abolishing the the City and County Development Boards (CDBs) and establishing Local Community Development Committees. The reform is envisaged to result in a more cohesive structure in place for coordinating economic and social development, whereby the work currently being done under the local authorities, CDBs and LEADER (rural development partnerships) groups will all join together under the new committees. Whether the new system will benefit local government community development work, remains to be seen.

Northern Ireland

The current system of local government

As with the way the system in the Republic was illustrated, the following section will demonstrate the fundamental structure of local government today, in terms of form (composition), functions, financial arrangement, and the reform and modernisation agenda. It is important to note that during various time periods since the foundation of the state in 1920, Northern Ireland's local government has provided its citizens with ongoing and much-needed democratic representation, especially the periods when direct rule from London was in place (Knox, 2003), and laid the foundation for the densely instituted community sector currently in place (Tonge, 2005). The people of Northern Ireland have associated political stability with the local government system, as it, unlike the mechanisms for central government devolved administrations, has never been abolished in favour of direct rule. District councils have, during the imposition of direct rule in Northern Ireland, been the only foci of local representation and democracy. The future of the local government system must balance the need for efficiency in the delivery of services, and the importance of the system in the daily lives of the Northern Irish people (Birrell and Hayes, 1999; Knox, 2003).

Form

Local government in Northern Ireland is made of up a single tier of councils, as a result of the Local Government (Northern Ireland) Act (1972) and the recommendations within the Macrory Report (1970). There are twenty-six district councils in Northern Ireland; operated by 582 councillors. However, as a result of the RPA process (initiated in 2002 and the results of which are contained within the strategy document *Better Government for Northern Ireland* (Northern Ireland Office, 2006)), reform of local government will see this number reduced from twenty-six to eleven, with the number of councillors reducing to 462, as clarified by a respondent within the Northern Ireland Local Government Association (NILGA). The process is set to be completed by April 2015 (Department of the Environment, 2013a).

Functions

The division of functions allocated to the authorities was less than those allocated in the local government systems across the UK. The Local Government (Transfer of Functions) (Northern Ireland) (1973) Act prescribed the functions, which can be divided into direct role, consultative role and representative role (Birrell and Hayes, 1999). The passing of the Northern Ireland Constitution Act (1973) abolished the Parliament of Northern Ireland, and the post of Governor (in place since 1921), and replaced the institutions with a devolved administration, made up of the Northern Ireland Assembly which would choose its own executive. The Act also delineated the division of functions in local government.

Direct role: the district councils in Northern Ireland are responsible for their own geographical location and the provision on services to the resident citizens (Birrell and Hayes, 1999). Sixty per cent of local government expenditure is spent on waste management, leisure and community services, street cleaning, recreation amenities and parks and open spaces. Some other important functions are regulatory in nature, and pertain to building control and environmental health functions. The regulatory role of councils has also been classified as part of the executive role of local authorities (Knox, 2003).

Consultative role: responsibilities in this regard relate to the authorities reflecting the opinions of their community. The district councils must be consulted on issues of regional importance to a particular council at any time

(Knox, 2003). The most developed consultative function is with the NIHE, which was established in 1971 (Birrell and Hayes, 1999). The district councils have the opportunity within this function to consult with central government departments on matters relating planning, development, roads and water services.

Representative role: as part of this role, local councillors sit on area boards, in order to ensure public representatives serve the needs of their communities on public agency boards, in the provision of state services (Knox, 2003).

Currently in relation to health functions, the councillor's role is representative rather than the council being responsible for service delivery, apart from some health promotion activity and communicable disease work (such as Legionnaires' disease outbreaks and assisting investigations into food poisoning). Councils are also consulted regarding major changes to health services in their area, as clarified by a respondent from NILGA during phase II of the study.

Finance

Spending by district councils accounts for less than 5 per cent of all public expenditure in Northern Ireland (Northern Ireland Executive, 2001; Knox, 2003), although this figure is rising. Local councils have three main sources of funding; district rate, the general grant and specific government grants (Knox, 2003). Northern Ireland is the only region in Ireland and Britain that administers the old system of property rates or taxes in financing local government (McKay, 1991). Services provided by local government are financed by the property tax system or rates. Both local and central government fix rates. Local councils set the district rate each year, and the tax base is made up of the 'rentable value of property (residential and business) or its net annual value' (Knox, 2003: 463).

Reform

The viewpoint exists that Northern Ireland suffers from saturated governance and representation (Birrell and Hayes, 1999; Knox, 2003; Knox and Carmichael, 2005). There are 101 Assembly members (MLAs) (central government) and 582 councillors (local government), representing a population of just under 1.84 million people (Northern Ireland Statistics and Research Agency, 2014a). John (1993) points out that an amalgamation of councils, in a bid to modernise the system in preparation for a transfer of more powers, would benefit the system overall. This is a recommendation of the RPA process also (Northern Ireland Office, 2006). Power-sharing has been a feature of local government politics over the past number of decades and would ease the reduction in the number of councils in line with this rationalisation agenda (Birrell and Hayes, 1999).

The reform programme in Northern Ireland aims to ensure that local government is at the heart of community life and service delivery (Wilford *et al.*, 2007). In order to achieve this, a reduction in the number of councils, from twenty-six to eleven, will be achieved by 2015. In 2006, a Local Government Reform Taskforce was established to ensure the process is well informed and is implemented smoothly. It is part of the central government's plan to transfer powers to local government once the larger councils have been established. One respondent within BCC in Northern Ireland summed up the reform process for local government:

> The local government council structure is going to have a whole improved service provision through new responsibilities and the whole range of broader powers and combined with partnership-working with central government agencies and with more consultation this is to make local authorities stronger, more effective, and flexible to local needs, avoid duplication, deliver more efficient high quality services.

This respondent stated that there was a 'plethora of activities ongoing' in order to achieve these structural changes by April 2015, and it was difficult to say exactly how the new structures would operate. The reform of local government would also involve a transfer of some of the planning and regeneration services and functions to the local authorities, which should also benefit instruments and approaches, such as HIA, towards building healthier public policies, as mentioned by local authority officials in an interview in phase II of the study.

In relation to functions of the local authorities, with the impeding implementation of the structural change of local authorities from 1 April 2015, the eleven new councils will take on the direct delivery role for planning, some roads functions – (mainly off-street car parking), some local economic development functions, regeneration and some housing functions (HMOs), and some other miscellaneous functions (respondent from NILGA).

As part of the reform programme, a new and innovative function of community planning will be performed by councils, to ensure joined-up governance between central and local tiers (Department of the Environment, 2013b). In relation to reform in Northern Ireland, community planning is defined as:

> a process led by councils in conjunction with partners and communities to develop and implement a shared vision for their area, a long term vision which relates to all aspects of community life and which also involves working together to plan and deliver better services which make a real difference to people's lives. (Department of the Environment, 2013b: 1)

This definition very much echoes the sentiment underlying the HIA ethos, in terms of its focus on partnership working and better informed and delivered plans and services. The Community Planning Foundation Programme has been developed as part of preparations for local government reform, to take place by April 2015. It is envisaged that the programme will assist Statutory

Transition Committees, the new councils and the community planning partners to prepare for community planning before the introduction of statutory community planning by April 2015 (Department of the Environment, 2013b). The Local Government Act (Northern Ireland) 2014 places the duty on local councils to initiate and facilitate a participative process for all partners in support of community planning. Government departments (ministries) will be required to support and promote community planning. Community plans will last for four years, and will be monitored by the councils and their partners.

Local government's public health roles: potential for increased partnership

The role of health within local government in RoI diminished greatly when the health functions were transferred to the Regional Health Boards under the Health Act 1970. Currently, the place of health within local authorities has been within the CDBs, this being the location of the Healthy City projects for the most part. However the authorities have no direct role in health and cooperate with the HSE and other agencies on matters of public health. In NI, as stated already, the authorities have a role in some health promotion and communicable disease activities, and the councils are consulted with regularly on any major changes connected to local health services. In both jurisdictions, neither local government system has direct health functions, however they do have a more consultative role in working on local public health agendas. This consultative role for public health and the alignment of local government work with local public health activities are some ways in which HIA and other HiAP endeavours could be further integrated with the local government systems.

The development of the health promotion and health improvement agenda in Northern Ireland and the Republic of Ireland

By 2012 the population of the Republic of Ireland stood at 4.6 million (Department of Health, 2012). Since 2003 population growth had increased by 15 per cent with population ageing also contributing to the growth (Department of Health, 2012). Life expectancy for men was 76.8 years and for women, 81.6 years (Department of Health, 2012: 9), exceeding the EU average by one year. The population of Northern Ireland stood at just under 1.84 million people in 2014 (Northern Ireland Statistics and Research Agency, 2014a). For the 2010 and 2012 period, life expectancy stood at 77.7 for men and 82.1 for women (Northern Ireland Statistics and Research Agency, 2014b). In Northern Ireland, the major causes of mortality and morbidity include circulatory and respiratory diseases and cancer (O'Neill *et al.*, 2012) while in the

Republic, diseases of the circulatory system are also the major causes of death and disease, as well as respiratory diseases, cancers and injuries (Department of Health, 2013). The main causes of death and disease do not differ hugely between both jurisdictions and concur with international trends for developed countries. Inequalities in health and social class continue to be a major predictor of disease rates (Department of Health, 2013). Non-communicable diseases account for the majority of deaths and disease. Interventions and key strategic actions are necessary to prevent and delay the onset of what are potentially preventable diseases (Institute of Public Health in Ireland, 2012). Health promotion and improvement activities in both NI and RoI account for the majority of interventions and strategic actions addressing risk factors for these major aforementioned diseases by adopting a determinants of health approach.

As part of the Belfast/Good Friday Agreement (1998) the North South Ministerial Council was set up, to develop consultation and cooperation on matters of mutual interest and competence. Health is one of the key areas in which the council has agreed to cooperate. It is from within this context that the all-island IPH was established. This was a major decision regarding the coordination and advancement of a cohesive public health agenda for the island of Ireland. The Institute of Public Health (IPH) is managed dually via the Belfast and Dublin offices. The rationale for establishing such an Institute was to facilitate greater cooperation and cohesiveness in coordinating a cross-border public health agenda, to the benefit of the island's citizens, professionals and policy-makers. The Institute is funded by the DHSSPS in Northern Ireland and the Department of Health in the Republic of Ireland. Three main areas of work include strengthening public health intelligence, building public health capacity, and policy and programme development and evaluation. The Institute is also involved in other all-island endeavours such as the Centre for Ageing Research Development in Ireland (CARDI), which it hosts. In relation to 'building public health capacity', the Institute is the leader in the promotion of healthier public policy through the use of HIA (Gillespie and McIldoon, 2009). It is an unrelenting champion of advancing HIA, and broadly the HiAP approach, in both jurisdictions.

In the Republic of Ireland, a number of key developments have occurred since the establishment of the Health Education Bureau in 1975 (Cahill, 2012). Since then, the international context for health promotion, influenced by the Ottawa Charter on Health Promotion (WHO, 1986), has shaped the health promotion agenda in the Republic of Ireland, as is the case in Northern Ireland also. Key developments include the establishment of the Health Promotion Unit in the Department of Health in 1988, the first Health Promotion Strategy (*Making the Healthier Choice, the Easier Choice*, 1995) and the subsequent strategy (*National Health Promotion Strategy 2000–2005*, 2000). Currently activities, which are statutorily coordinated and delivered through the HSE, are guided by the *Health Promotion Strategic Framework* (2011). The new national framework for action to improve health and wellbeing, *Healthy Ireland – Framework for Improved Health and Well-being, 2013 to 2025* (Department of Health, 2013) seeks to address health inequalities, improve health protection, create supportive environments and take action appropriately using a life-course approach.

The Health Promotion Agency (HPA) Northern Ireland was the body responsible for coordinating and delivering health promotion plans and actions. The HPA was one body that had this responsibility and had a very specific role at a regional level while the local commissioners of the four health and social care boards had the local responsibility and would have been more active in communities. The HPA was set up in 1990 as an agency of the DHSSPS and was accountable to the Minister responsible for Health. The *Investing for Health* strategy (2002) embodied the strategic aims and objectives of the Health Promotion Agency. In reality the strategy was much broader than this and indeed HPA would have been one of the bodies charged with implementation along with the four boards with the latter bodies having taken forward the bulk of the work. *Investing for Health* has been Northern Ireland's strategy to promote public health and wellbeing. It was launched in response to the previous Executive's commitment to population health and life expectancy improvements. The most recent public health framework strategy *Making Life Better* was announced and launched in 2014. It builds on the work of *Investing for Health* in terms of addressing the risk factors for many of the preventable diseases (Institute of Public Health in Ireland, 2012). Since 1 April 2009 responsibilities and tasks of the Health Promotion Agency and the four health and social care boards have been transferred to the PHA, specifically and mostly to the Health and Social Wellbeing Improvement section. This is outlined by a respondent from the PHA:

> The functions of the Health Promotion Agency (HPA) were absorbed into the new PHA, along with the functions of public health of the four health and social care boards, and the four Investing for Health partnerships and staff, and the four health action zones. Within health and social wellbeing improvement, you had 13 organisations amalgamate under the PHA, and the HPA was one of 13 organisations that came to together, and the change, was in relation to how they relate to one another and their direct functions.

Health promotion through the medium of television, radio and public information campaigns come under the Community and Knowledge Management Operations of the PHA. All activities being coordinated by the Health and Social Wellbeing Improvement section are those which fell previously under the responsibility of the Health Promotion Agency and legacy boards. This has been as part of the reorganisation reform agenda initiated as part of the RPA.

Having explored the different structural and statutory contexts for HIA activity, the following section examines the way in which HIA has developed, and continues to advance, across the island of Ireland.

HIA development across the Republic of Ireland and Northern Ireland

Already we have seen in this chapter the governance structure and context of local government, and the way that the health systems are structured and managed, according to government-led priorities. Both systems in both jurisdictions are in the process of change at the time of writing, which makes this an interesting time to explore a policy-informing instrument such as HIA. In Northern Ireland, the RPA still is having a major impact on the day-to-day work of officials, all of which will become clearer by April 2015 when the changes are planned to be fully implemented. The amalgamation of local authorities in Northern Ireland means that many officials are yet to meet their new colleagues and directors, all of whom need to be in place by April 2015. This is a major change and challenge to the daily and strategic working at a local government level, and also in the public health system which is equally subject to the RPA process of reform. This state of fluctuation in itself impacts the conduct of HIAs as, for example, new personnel in the local authorities and in the PHA will often not be aware of HIA and perhaps, therefore, not open to being involved in one, as raised by a respondent from the PHA in phase II of the study's data collection. The restructuring of the systems means also a movement of personnel around to new sections and offices, which can very often result in a loss of experience and expertise in using, or being familiar at least, with the HIA approach. This is where legislation for HIA would prevent such loss of knowledge; if it were mainstreamed, such expertise would not be lost so easily and so ineffectually. In the Republic of Ireland, the local government system is undergoing many changes as part of a reform programme. A major impact of this on HIA is the abolishment of the CDBs, which currently hosts the Healthy City projects (which in turn work to advance HIA amongst other associated priorities). This means that Healthy City projects are in a state of flux and uncertainty as to where they sit within the local authority, as raised by a respondent from the HSE in phase II of the study's data collection. CDBs will be incorporated into Local Enterprise Offices (LEOs), but until this happens (after the local elections of 23 May 2014), local authorities, which are the WHO-designated hosts to the Healthy City projects, may be at the very least unsure as to how to advance the projects and their actions.

In the Republic of Ireland, at the time of writing, the WHO-designated Healthy Cities include Cork, Galway and Waterford, and in Northern Ireland include Derry/Londonderry and Belfast. A National Network of Healthy Cities in Ireland has been set up within the Republic so as to bring together the experiences of the projects and enable a sharing of knowledge of the Healthy Cities in the country. The Healthy City projects in Northern Ireland are included and represented within the UK Healthy City Network, although there will also be communication of experiences and activities on an all-island basis amongst the five city projects in the Healthy Cities Network Ireland, as highlighted by a respondent from the HSE management in phase II of the study's data collection. This follows the approach of many public health endeavours on the island being coordinated on an all-island basis, to facilitate cohesive partnership working, knowledge-sharing and collaboration across the two jurisdictions. The Belfast Healthy Cities Partnership (BHC) celebrated its twenty-fifth anniversary in 2013, which is a significant milestone. BHC acts as a leader in promoting a HiAP approach across policy sectors in Northern Ireland and in advancing and promoting HIA. The partnership is also a leading member of the WHO European Healthy Cities Network. BHC has much experience and a proven track record in working to improve health equity and wellbeing for people living and working in Belfast city. For both jurisdictions, BHC is a body that stands as a beacon in terms of what can be achieved within the workings of a Healthy City project.

A common denominator in the development of the HIA agenda in both jurisdictions is the role of the Institute of Public Health, which collaborates across the border in order to ensure capacity and knowledge is shared on HIA in a cohesive and coordinated manner. This is to the great benefit of HIA's advancement and future as a policy-aiding instrument and approach. The IPH has been identified as 'the primary provider of HIA support services and advocacy' (Gillespie and McIldoon, 2009: 40) in the Republic of Ireland and in Northern Ireland as identified in a review conducted of HIA activity by the IPH in the years 2001 to 2009. Difficulties with implementing HIA were identified at strategic and operational levels, which refer to the lack of resources and the lack of a legislative basis for implementing HIA, and 'the mechanisms/structures for delivering HIAs on a wide scale are not in place' in either jurisdiction (Gillespie and McIldoon, 2009: 40).

In terms of planning services and environmental protection, in Northern Ireland it will be interesting to examine HIAs' role alongside the Community Planning proposal within the Local Government Act (Northern Ireland) 2014, to come into force by 2015. In both jurisdictions, planning services being operated at the local authority level are already dealing with a planning system that is cumbersome and somewhat overloaded with regulations and requirements, and for a local authority to conduct or even be involved in a HIA, without a legislative base for the approach and instrument, is a challenge. The lack of legislative basis of HIA in both jurisdictions does mean it is less secure in its place as an instrument and approach in promoting healthier public policy. One way of ensuring that HIA, or even the consideration of health impacts, is more embedded within the system is to incorporate it into an IIA, or Policy Toolkit, as is in place in Northern Ireland at the Assembly level. It also could be amalgamated with EIA or SEA. In the Republic of Ireland according to the *Healthy Ireland* national framework, HIA is proposed to be strengthened within the licensing structure by the EPA in order to further integrate and improve health considerations in environmental protection activities. However how this will be implemented in reality remains to be seen.

Notably in both jurisdictions, HIA within the national policy documents and frameworks for public health and health promotion (namely, *Healthy Ireland* 2013 (RoI); *Health Promotion Strategic Framework* 2011 (RoI); and the public health framework for Northern Ireland *Making Life Better* 2014) has been very much diluted in terms of its role in contributing to advancing a holistic public health agenda in promoting population health and healthier public policies. This is in stark contrast to the supportive wording and strong statements regarding HIA in the previous major policy documents.

One of the key objectives within the Health Strategy *Quality and Fairness: A Health System for You* (RoI) (Department of Health and Children, 2001: 61) was the importance of locating population health within the remit of public policy development.

The strategy identifies HIA as an integral policy-proofing tool, as defined in the following:

> (It is) a means for all sectors to determine the effects of their policies and actions on health and it has the potential to bring greater transparency to the decision-making process by clarifying the nature of trade-offs in policy. (Department of Health and Children, 2001: 61)

The strategy states that 'HIA will be introduced as part of the public policy development process' (Department of Health and Children, 2001: 157) at all tiers of governance structures. This is a prophetic and bold call for this policy-proofing instrument to be institutionalised within Irish policy-making circles. The strategy states that the Department of Health and Children is identified as having the main responsibility in ensuring HIAs are implemented and supported throughout the system. Regional and local level structures, such as local authorities and CDBs, are to be encouraged in assimilating HIAs within the policy process. The importance of ensuring HIAs are conducted at local level is emphasised throughout the Health Strategy.

Fast-forward approximately twelve years and this bold language and statement on HIA is not reflected in the same way in the later *Healthy Ireland* (2013) policy framework. Rather, within *Healthy Ireland*, SIA is promoted as the tool which will be implemented at the local level and which will incorporate poverty impact assessment and 'health impacts will be a core feature of this new tool' (Department of Health, 2013: 13). One respondent interviewed for this book, from the Institute of Public Health, stated the following in relation to *Healthy Ireland* and the place of HIAs within it:

> the aspirations of HIA fairly (are)enshrined in that intent to assess the impact of the effect of public policy on population health, but the explicit references to HIA don't exist (in *Healthy Ireland*), what they refer to is a methodology of SIA which encompasses dimensions of health, that is the tool to try and ensure a whole of government approach brings a social determinants and health inequalities approach.

Certainly there is an identified change in how HIA is envisioned over the next period of time, compared with the goals of the 2001 and 2002 strategies in RoI and NI. One may say that once the health impacts of projects, programmes and policies are being assessed systematically within an instrument or approach, then the label we give to that tool (IIA, SIA or HIA) is not as important as the work being done in promoting improved social and health wellbeing, as the respondent went on to say:

> It depends, does that really matter for me, the fact that it's not stated explicitly or that the outcomes of successful HIA are addressed through other methodologies (such as SIA) … is it a stumbling block or barrier, is that really there, or are people taking a health lens to the development of their policy, and that is enough.

All will be revealed as to the implementation in reality of these tools and instruments in the future, and the extent to which the assessment of health impacts will have a significant role to play within SIA. The incorporation of health impacts into the Policy Toolkit in Northern Ireland Assembly is quite significant, 'there is a lot of emphasis on health' in that Toolkit, which provides a useful lesson for the development of SIA hopefully. The Department of Social Protection will lead on developing the SIA toolkit with input from the Institute of Public Health which has vast experience in developing and training in the HIA tool in the Republic of Ireland and Northern Ireland. The Health Strategy 2001 promised that HIA would be introduced as part of the public policy development process at all tiers of governance structures (which it was not on a systematic basis) and that support would come from the Department of Health and Children (later renamed Department of Health) in implementing HIA (which can be said it is doing indirectly through the support and training provided by the Institute of Public Health). When questioned as to why HIA has been diluted, a respondent from the Institute of Public Health stated that the lack of a legislative basis for HIA slowed down its institutionalisation and also since it did not become a defined part of work for individuals in the Department of Health or DHSSPS, it has not been taken on board so much:

> If it doesn't have any recognition of its capacity, capability, potential at the highest level, if it doesn't have a legislative base or isn't enshrined in someone's work profile or business plan, it often falls to the enthusiastic individual to champion its implementation, it's similar in Northern Ireland and the Republic of Ireland,

> in the absence of those particulars it's difficult for it to be sustained or maintained in a systemic manner.

Also, political philosophy was identified as a hurdle to the wider HiAP agenda and the determinants of health approaches, as mentioned by one respondent working within the HSE. That is to say, that the political philosophy embodied within governing structures, local and national, are often not familiar with the wider determinants of health and are still focused on individualised interventions to address public health issues as opposed to adopting a more holistic focus on health whereby healthier public policies and a wider determinants of health approach would better address and tackle health inequalities and facilitate health improvement.

It is not only HIA that is changing its format, as the changing nature of health promotion terminology within *Healthy Ireland* (2013) and within the restructuring of the HSE is also clear. A similar trend has been happening in Northern Ireland also within the Health and Social Wellbeing Improvement Directorate under the PHA. The change in the wording of health promotion activities to health improvement is reflective of the way the field changes names and labels for activities rather than a significant move away from the main tenets of work involved in the promotion and protection of public health. This issue was raised during discussions with respondents from the PHA.

In Northern Ireland, in the new public health framework *Making Life Better*, the statement and support of HIA is not as strong as it was in the 2002 *Investing for Health* strategy, although is not as diluted as much as has happened in the comparable *Healthy Ireland*:

> A similar process to develop a public health framework in Northern Ireland (has been happening), so that again, going back to *Investing for Health*, there was a whole chapter on HIA, it's a dilution in the explicit references to HIA as a method to achieving healthy public policy. (Respondent from the Institute of Public Health)

The policy document *Investing for Health* (2002) has been Northern Ireland's strategy to promote public health and wellbeing. It was launched in response to the previous Executive's commitment to population health and life expectancy improvements. In order to achieve the aims and goals of the strategy, *Investing for Health* (2002: 172) outlines the rationale for HIA:

> The success of much of the proposed agenda for action will depend on the impacts of all Department's policies and programmes. HIAs of non-health policies are increasingly seen as a key tool to facilitate cross-sectoral action, and to promote health and reduce inequalities.

The DHSSPS is the leading agency in promoting the use of HIA whilst coordinating action in the area with the all-island Institute of Public Health and

Department of Health and Children in the Republic. The promotion of HIA in Northern Ireland will occur in an incremental manner, in order to address 'issues of coordination, capacity building, tool development and quality assurance' (2002). The DHSSPS was to coordinate action with other government ministries in order to support the institutionalisation of the tool, which it appears to have been doing according to the review of the strategy (FGS McClure Watters Consulting, 2010). Mapping of policy formulation cycles and health policies in non-health sectors is one of the goals of the leading health department in the strive for institutionalisation of HIAs. The integration of HIA with an all-encompassing IIA tool is an identified option for the way forward for HIA, as well within the SEA, which was implemented in 2004. This integration happened to some extent with the Policy Toolkit, developed by the OFMDFM. The review of the *Investing for Health* strategy (FGS McClure Watters Consulting, 2010: 11) states that the department continues to promote HIA as a 'tool to facilitate cross-sectoral action and to promote and reduce inequalities'. The report also states that 'consideration should also be given to a mandatory requirement for all Departments to conduct HIAs and/or the HiAP approach in their policy development processes', however, as in the RoI, nothing has been done in terms of legislation for the HIA instrument and approach. In Northern Ireland, however, the impact of the RPA will not be truly known until after the changes have been implemented, in terms of restructuring from April 2015 onwards. For now, based on current policy frameworks, the HIA instrument and approach is not as strongly promoted as it was early in the 2000s.

Conclusion: similarities and differences

This chapter introduced and outlined the systems of health and of local government that are in place in both jurisdictions which HIA must engage with when being planned, conducted and monitored. At the Fifth Global Conference on Health Promotion, HIA was advocated as a 'key activity required to promote healthy policymaking at the local level', which could stimulate action and generate tangible results (Mittelmark, 2000: 14). The local level is often seen as more conducive for the conduct of HIAs than the national level (Davenport *et al.*, 2006). However one respondent in the Institute of Public Health stated that although HIAs in both jurisdictions are conducted primarily at the local level, often it is 'in spite of, instead of because of, local structures … HIAs are being done at local level but there are no structures aiding the conduct of HIAs'. The respondent referred to the fact that HIA is not specifically within anyone's job description at these levels currently and it is, more often than not, up to the enthusiastic champions of the approach to use and advance HIA. This is why it is vital that high level political leadership especially supports local government and governance structures and health system structures at national and local levels in the promotion of healthier public policy through the embedding of instruments and approaches such as HIA, which can lead to a whole-of-government approach to addressing population health and wellbeing. Often the work and role of the individual champion for the HIA approach and instrument in advancing a healthier public policy and HiAP approach is still a determining factor in the use of such approaches.

The local government level was identified as a strategic and appropriate level for HIAs to be conducted in Ireland as noted by a HIA practitioner (Ison, 2007, cited in Kearns and Pursell, 2007: 55):

> Local government works with all sectors, employs people from many disciplines, deals with inequalities in its population, collects both quantitative and qualitative data, and has experience in community consultation and participation. This … makes the local government value base complementary to that of HIA, given its focus on sustainability, its democratic character, and its concern to reduce inequity.

Both jurisdictions have similar challenges to face in relation to the local government systems which are in the process of structural changes and in the health system structures also. Both jurisdictions have similar public health frameworks which are developed at similar time periods (2013 and 2014), both of which mention HIA only implicitly as an instrument and approach to facilitate healthier public policies, which is a big change when compared to similar policy strategies of 2001 (Health Strategy, Republic of Ireland) and 2002 (*Investing for Health*, Northern Ireland) which called boldly for action around HIA institutionalisation. Gillespie and McIldoon (2009) recommended that the Department of Health in the Republic of Ireland reviews its responsibilities as outlined in the *Quality and Fairness* strategy (Health Strategy) (2001) and in Northern Ireland that the DHSSPS must review its responsibilities to HIA under *Investing for Health*, and should ensure that HIA is included on the agenda of the Ministerial Group on Public Health (MGPH). The change in emphasis on HIA in the more recent policy frameworks does not inspire confidence that HIA will be prioritised in the future. However, whether HIA needs to be present in name, or can exist within approaches and tools such as the SIA, other IAs, and HiAP approaches, remains to be seen. Reasons identified for the dilution of HIA, at least explicitly, are connected to its lack of a legislative base, the fact that it is often not within the remit of public health or local government officials' job description to conduct or refer to HIA work, and notably the fact that high level political endorsement is missing for the HIA instrument and approach. The hope is that, within the structures that will arise as a result of key changes in the local government and health service sectors, HIA can find a home, as Kearns and Pursell (2007: 56) noted, 'given the potential benefits of HIA from a public health perspective, it is imperative that managers, policy and decision makers in both the Irish the local government and health sectors engage with the relevant stakeholders in community, voluntary and academic communities in the development, conduct and evaluation of HIA.' This can apply to both jurisdictions.

In the following chapter, HIAs with a focus on the physical environment are examined, whilst Chapter 5 examines HIAs conducted on housing plans and programmes. These HIAs provide the necessary 'real world' feel for the instrument and approach that can be lost when examining policy documents only. They will illustrate the ways in which HIA can inform (or not) local policy development.

Note

1 The author would like to thank and acknowledge the invaluable comments and information of Brendan Bonner, Aodh Quinlivan and Karen Smyth on this chapter.

4

HIA in the physical environment

Policy development and community participation

This chapter commences with a brief overview of the population health impacts of the physical environment. Two HIAs are then described and explored using the conceptual lens as outlined in Chapter 2. This chapter describes HIAs conducted in the area of the physical environment; one on traffic and transport and the other is on a Draft Air Quality Action Plan. The initiatives and plans that the HIAs were conducted on arose from the local authority (respectively, DCC and BCC). A background description is given of each HIA (how and why they came about) and the story behind the HIA is elaborated. As a result of the analysis of interviews conducted with participants on the HIA steering committees/groups representing all key stakeholders in the years 2007 and 2008 (local authority, community, public health, HIA experts and other local agencies) (phase I of the study), each HIA includes an exploration of the perspectives of the individuals sitting on each HIA's steering committees. An update of the impact of the HIAs is provided also as a result of a follow-up examination carried out in 2013 and 2014 (phase II of the study).

Physical environment and health impacts

It is well accepted that the living space in terms of the physical and social environment is a determinant on the health and wellbeing of individuals, communities and societies across the world (Frumkin *et al.*, 2004). In 2006 the Institute of Public Health published *Health Impacts of the Built Environment: A Review*, which outlines and highlights how buildings, public spaces and social networks have direct impacts on population health and wellbeing (Lavin *et al.*, 2006). A number of studies have examined the linkages between health and the physical environment, such as the impacts of pedestrian-friendly designs on air pollution exposure (De Nazelle *et al.*, 2009); active transport initiative and youth physical activity (Grow *et al.*, 2008); and the effect of the physical environment on mental wellbeing (Cooper *et al.*, 2009; Taylor *et al.*, 2015).

Part of the physical environment within which we live includes the flow of traffic and transport (Douglas *et al.*, 2007). Boldo *et al.* (2011) conducted an HIA of a reduction in air pollution levels in Spain, concluding that general mortality would improve if pollution control policies were successfully implemented. The health impacts of transport and traffic on human health and wellbeing is well-documented, in Ireland (Kelly and Clancy, 1984; Clancy *et al.*, 2002; Kavanagh *et al.*, 2005) and internationally (Acheson, 1998; Marmot and Wilkinson, 1999; Douglas *et al.*, 2007; Geelen *et al.*, 2013). This overview is just that, a very brief overview of the wealth of scientific evidence demonstrating causal linkages between the physical environment around us, ranging from the built environment, air quality measures, the impact of transport and traffic, to name a few, and overall health and wellbeing. The overwhelming consensus is that, where you live and the space around you, will impact on your health and wellbeing, as the following section reflects in relation to the HIAs conducted on traffic and transport in RoI and on air quality in NI.

HIA on traffic and transport, 2004 (Dublin, Republic of Ireland)

Part I: description

A comprehensive retrospective HIA was carried out in 2003 and 2004 on transport initiatives in Ballyfermot, Dublin. Ballyfermot is situated within the boundary of DCC, located in the south central area. The HIA steering group involved a number of key stakeholders (statutory, community and advisory). A mixed method design was used in this impact assessment employing both qualitative and quantitative techniques. This is the first HIA carried out in either jurisdiction relating to traffic and transport of an inner city community.

The purpose of this HIA was to assess the air pollution levels in Ballyfermot and to investigate its impact upon the local populace. Transport initiatives ongoing in the area were looked at within the context of the process, focusing on their success in reducing traffic in the area. The choice of Ballyfermot was deemed an appropriate one by the advocates of the HIA project. The area was a designated socio-economically disadvantaged community with a poor physical environment (Hayes, 2003). Measures that would be put in place to reduce the levels of traffic would benefit the community at large. These initiatives were also believed to improve the social capital in the area and were envisaged to empower the resident stakeholders to take control of an issue directly affecting the community (Eastern Regional Health Authority (ERHA), 2004).

The aim of the process was to carry out an HIA on local authority transport initiatives in the Ballyfermot area and to then use the findings to achieve the following objectives:

- Influence the delivery of future transport policies and safety initiatives in the community.
- Inform the second review of the DCC Road Safety Plan.
- Provide a health focus to the Air Quality and Noise Assessment Project being conducted concurrently by DCC and funded by URBAN II.
- Influence the resource allocation for future health service delivery in Ballyfermot. (ERHA, 2004: 4)

The HIA was also expected to improve cross-sectoral collaboration on matters of health and physical exercise; to promote understanding across the various sectors of the link between transport and health status; to engage the community in active decision-making and to enable various sectors (statutory, voluntary and community) to work in partnership; and to enhance learning in the area of HIA (Hayes, 2003). More specifically, the terms of reference of the HIA were:

> to assess the health impacts of traffic elements of the Ballyfermot Village Plan, and the health impacts of the transport infrastructure support under the National Development Plan (NDP). (Hayes, 2006)

The Ballyfermot Village Plan (led and developed by DCC) includes the following initiatives: (1) traffic calming measures – ramps and speed cushions; (2) traffic islands and pedestrian refuge areas; (3) road signage and traffic light installations; (4) construction of designated bus and cycle lanes. Within the terms of reference it was specified that the HIA Merseyside Guidelines would be used as a standardised methodological framework for conducting the HIA (Scott-Samuel *et al.*, 2001).

Stakeholder involvement

A number of stakeholders participated on the steering group of the HIA. The following provides an overview of the main groups of stakeholders. A variety of participants from the steering group were interviewed in 2007 and 2008, and contact was re-made in 2014 with a selection of respondents. In this Ballyfermot HIA case study, eleven people were interviewed in phase I of the study (2007 and 2008) and four in 2014 (phase II).

The statutory health services

The Department of Public Health in the ERHA was successful in the tender for a HIA on traffic and transport in Ballyfermot in 2003, to the project funders, URBAN II. A steering group was established to manage and lead the HIA and ensure all stages, from literature review through data collection, were kept on schedule and in accordance with the outlined objectives. This committee consisted of representatives from the health services including the health services

(ERHA and the South Western Area Health Board (SWAHB) (currently the HSE)), URBAN II, residents from the local community who would be affected by initiatives in the area, the Institute of Public Health, DCC (including planning and traffic officials and engineers) and an external HIA consultant. The wide variety of stakeholders indicates the nature of the multi-sectoral dimension of the HIA in transport and traffic.

The health services were to play an integral role in the HIA both in terms of its planning, conduct, management and dissemination of findings. On the steering group there were four members representing the health services.

Dublin City Council

DCC is the local government authority governing the area of Ballyfermot. It was vital that officials from the council were present on the HIA, as many of the recommendations would require action and decision-making at the local authority level, albeit they were not obliged to undertake the HIA's recommendations due to a lack of legislative basis of HIA in the jurisdiction. Both the health services and the council were identified as the key decision-makers in the HIA report (ERHA, 2004). Four members from the council were present on the HIA steering group. One member of the Dublin Transportation Office was also present. DCC has decentralised its offices from Wood Quay in the city centre to various areas in the Dublin suburbs. The council officials working in the area are based in the Ballyfermot Civic Centre.

URBAN II

URBAN II was the Community Initiative of the ERDF for sustainable development in disadvantaged urban areas in the EU for the time period 2000 to 2006. URBAN II seeks to promote the implementation of innovative models of development for the economic and social redevelopment and regeneration of urban communities. The project advocates cross-country learning of experiences through the European network of cities and partners (Dublin City Council, 2001). In 2000 Ballyfermot's priorities for action were identified through community consultation. The Traffic and Transport HIA (2004) fit into these areas of action (URBAN, 2002). Since 2001, Ballyfermot URBAN staff and the local community worked together to bring about sustainable projects in order to initiate positive change. DCC is the local authority with responsibility to oversee the work of the programme in Ballyfermot. An important contextual factor for the URBAN II programme in Ireland is the nature of local government reform. Such reforms in Ireland aim to 'maximise local democratic influence on the local decision making process (which included at the time) the establishing of Strategic Policy Committees and Area Committees' (URBAN, 2002: 6). URBAN II involved the collaboration of local stakeholders and actors within the new framework of working in local government. Members of the Area Committee (elected representatives) have a key role in the democratic accountability of the work of the programme. Quinn (2007) reiterates this message of enhancing public consultation for local government. URBAN II in Ballyfermot completed its work by September 2008. The RAPID office in the Ballyfermot area office took over some responsibilities and activities of the URBAN II project.

RAPID, Ballyfermot Area Office

The RAPID programme is a central government strategy introduced in 2001. At the time of writing, there are fifty-one RAPID areas in the RoI (Pobal, 2014). In 2006 an evaluation of the RAPID programme was published for the then Department of Community, Rural and Gaeltacht Affairs. It emphasised the importance of community participation in local partnership processes, and identified the 'lack of success in empowering the community to influence the decision-making process' (cited in Community Workers Cooperative, 2006). The HIA in Ballyfermot was hoped to engage the community so as to ensure they would have a meaningful role in the local area decision-making processes. The Ballyfermot RAPID programme attained full status in 2007 and is integral to the collective activity of the community. The RAPID project was integral to the continuation of the HIA working group (known locally as the Impact Group) in order to maintain sustainability of the community action that was initiated within the HIA in 2004. There was no member of RAPID on the steering group of the HIA; however the project is integral to the sustainability of the HIA's work.

Community representatives

Local community representatives were a distinct and important actor on the HIA steering group. The HIA methodology advocates the importance of the involvement of community members (residents in this HIA) who would be affected by the policy decisions that the impact assessment process is aiming to influence. As was derived from data collection and interviews with the steering group members, they played a vital role in maintaining the HIA group at local level amongst residents. They were also involved in a field trip to Italy as part of dissemination of the HIA findings to other European partners.

External consultant/HIA expert

An external consultant was hired to provide practical skills and research expertise to the HIA process. This person is involved in the field of HIA, both in terms of academic and practical experience of the approach and technique.

Institute of Public Health (IPH)
The Institute of Public Health is an all-island agency which is based in Dublin and Belfast. On the steering group IPH members held advisory and supportive roles, as well as being instrumental in undertaking parts of the HIA process.

HIA methodology

A comprehensive retrospective HIA was conducted in Ballyfermot. A concurrent or prospective impact assessment was not viable, as the measures proposed by DCC relating to traffic and transport in the area were already decided upon by the time the HIA commenced. It was hoped therefore that the HIA would inform ongoing activities and future plans and initiatives. The Merseyside Guidelines for carrying out a HIA were adhered to, overseen and led by the steering group (Scott-Samuel *et al.*, 1998).

Data was collected for the impact assessment by using both qualitative and quantitative research methods, including focus groups with residents, interviews with key informants such as teachers, Gardaí Síochána (RoI state police) and health workers, and a quantitative review of data related to the health status of Ballyfermot residents, and a review of data of levels of traffic in the area, and a literature review of evidence relating to health and traffic, including a review of transport/traffic HIAs already conducted.

The findings from the data collection were collated and triangulated with evidence from the literature and other information relevant to the HIA. In this instance, findings from the Ballyfermot Air Quality and Noise Assessment were used during this stage (Dublin City Council, 2004). An 'appraisal day' was held to identify a number of recommendations for future traffic-related policy decisions for the Ballyfermot area. The stage following this appraisal involved the steering group communicating the provisional findings from the HIA to the Ballyfermot community. The individuals involved in the interviews, focus groups and key representatives of the community were involved in this feedback stage.

HIA outcomes (ERHA, 2004)

An evaluation report of this HIA was published in 2007 (Kearns and Pursell, 2007), three years after the completion of the project. This appraisal provides evidence as to the achievement of the proposed aims and objectives of the IA process. It was hoped that although the HIA had been completed too late to be considered in the DCC Road Safety Plan, the HIA would be utilised in the upcoming Road Safety Plan by DCC. After correlation of quantitative data collected in the HIA with the air quality assessment carried out by the DCC as the same time, it was concluded that air pollution levels were within international standards. Lifestyle behaviours of residents in the community, particularly smoking, were identified as risk factors more likely to damage the health of residents than environmental air pollution. However, the HIA outcome report did specify that monitoring of air pollution levels needed to be maintained in order to sustain the healthy situation in Ballyfermot and surrounding areas.

The HIA process uncovered numerous health issues, in particular the extent of health inequalities within the community. Ballyfermot, and all disadvantaged communities, are prioritised in terms of resource provision and health services. The assessment of need and health status, derived as part of the IA process, was used by the local area health board at the time (SWAHB).

An intangible and yet vital outcome of the HIA process was the extent of the intersectoral cooperation and partnership on matters relating to health and transport. In addition, the involvement of URBAN II was hoped to give the findings of the HIA a wider European audience. URBAN II is a European-wide project and dissemination of findings from individual countries' projects is one of the features of the initiative. It was identified by the steering group that the involvement of the Institute of Public Health was integral to the success of the project, in terms of dissemination of the project's findings, and as an integral network of statutory, voluntary and community groups on the island of Ireland.

It is standard practice that specific recommendations would be proposed at the conclusion of a HIA process, which was the case in this instance.

Policy process for the Ballyfermot HIA

It was the aim of the HIA steering group that findings of the process would be used by DCC in its Road Safety Plan and City Development Plans, by the HSE in the formulation of tailored health services for the community, and more broadly by the Department of Transport as part of the National Development Plan (central government roadmap for growth and development in the RoI). In reality, it has informed HSE health promotion initiatives and policy development at local authority level, although more implicitly than explicitly for DCC. It was cited as a key source of evidence by a locally elected representative to DCC.

Part II: analysis

Interviews conducted with respondents for this HIA case were analysed and the results of this analysis are presented in the following section. The conceptual lens, as outlined in Chapter 2, provides a framework for presenting the findings from the interview data. As already mentioned, in this Ballyfermot HIA case study, eleven people were interviewed in phase I of the study (2007 and 2008) and four in 2014 (phase II).

'Institutions matter': New Institutional Theory

As discussed in Chapter 2, the normative dimension in New Institutional Theory alludes to the norms within institutions that can go some way to explain the behaviour of actors in the institutions and organisations. It is from this normative institutionalism that the 'major comeback' of the New Institutionalist approach made its way (Peters, 1999). March and Olsen's seminal work (1984; 1989; 1995) puts forward the idea that the behaviour of individuals must be explained and explored within normative principles; individual action being constrained or enabled by the institutional setting and the norms, standards and processes that come from that environment. The influence of the institution, and its norms, has been cited in previous HIA policy research, as a further explanatory theory to allow the exploration of the influences upon the use of HIAs in policy (Banken, 2001; 2003; Bekker *et al.*, 2005; Kemm, 2005; Bekker, 2007; Morgan, 2008). Therefore for this study, institutional influence was explored and discussed with the respondents.

A number of questions were asked during the interviews, so as to explore the degree of influence institutional norms had in the use of the HIA report, and the knowledge that came from that and its preceding process. The responses and discussions that arose from the interviews in relation to this idea are presented in the following section.

Are institutions ready? The timing of HIA as a policy support instrument and approach

The timing of HIA as a policy support instrument and approach was asked about so as to explore the perspective of those in the HIA steering group which included both decision-makers of statutory bodies and the community perspective. Five of those interviewed stated that yes, the time was right in our policy-making world for HIA to influence and thus inform policy. These individuals came from the community, health services and the local authority. Two respondents were more sceptical of the process, stating 'maybe'; they believed there were a number of possible constraining factors that might inhibit the incorporation and use of HIAs in policy, such as time and workload limitations and a lack of legislative basis for HIA. One individual from the local authority stated that no, the time had not come for HIAs to be used in the policy process, as is further illustrated in the following quotation:

> It's (HIA) a useful exercise in gathering statistics but not sure what changes have come from the study apart from a number of recommendations. This HIA has not paved the way, I don't think so.

Despite this perspective of the Ballyfermot HIA process and the impact it can have on the policy process, the overall sentiment of the steering group was that the time had come for knowledge and evidence from HIAs to be used to influence policy-making.

Normative dimension: do institutions shape behaviour?
The use of institutional theory in this study allows for an exploration of the extent of the influence that certain institutions have in the use of HIAs and the knowledge that came from them which was intended to inform policy, both in the short and long term. Those interviewed from this HIA were stakeholders in the process and were on the steering group as representatives for their respective institutional bodies.

The HIA was promoted and led by members within the health services sector. One leading individual from within the sector reflected that although the progress of HIAs was still at an early stage of learning and development, the policy of the HSE was to promote and advocate its growth and use. This individual was also a key member of the HIQA, working on the HIA agenda in conjunction with the IPH. This was a promising development at the time. However since the time of this interview in 2007, the HSE service plan currently (in 2014) does not have an explicit policy to promote and advocate HIAs, as discussed in Chapter 3 (interviews with respondents from the HSE and Institute of Public Health). Kearns and Pursell (2007) concluded that the instrument being embedded within the health services was a necessary requirement if HIAs were to be mainstreamed and used on a systematic basis to inform policy, both within and outside, the health services. However despite this recommendation, this has not happened since 2007, and instead it remains to be seen if health impacts of projects, programmes and policies will be adequately considered within the SIA tool as advocated within the current *Healthy Ireland* (2013) public health framework in place, as was discussed in Chapter 3.

The importance of local authorities having a central role, both on HIA steering groups, and in the use of HIA evidence, was highlighted in the interviews. One respondent from the health services said that 'the local authority need to come on board, what's needed is a top-down approach from them'. This highlights the necessity of having the main decision-making bodies involved in the HIA process, and at least awareness of the processes ongoing, as they are the institutions to directly use the health impacts knowledge in policy. However the lack of legislative obligation on local authorities or any statutory bodies to undertake and use HIAs is missing, which makes the use of HIA knowledge much more challenging.

Institutional structures of the different bodies, however, can be a barrier to the development of HIA, as is indicated in the following statement by one senior official in the local authority:

> Different organisations would have control over budgets, might not be doing the same thing on Steering Group, not all doing the same aim, difficult to pull all together, HSE budgets and local authority separately implement with coordinating committees. That can be a problem.

The different agendas and interests of the varying institutions which are brought to the table can inhibit the progress of the HIA, although this can be negated by a clarification of such issues at the beginning of the process, as suggested by one individual from the local authority.

Another local authority respondent also stated that an 'institution has to be persuaded of the benefits of HIA, so that it's not a philosophical exercise'. When asked to clarify this statement, the individual went on to say, 'I mean that it's too academic focused, not outcome focused'. This indicates the view that HIA must ensure it fits the expectations, requirements and norms of the institutions that are represented within its process, and will use it, in the short and long term. This 'institutionalisation' of HIAs, by becoming embedded in processes and procedures by aligning itself with such norms, is an important step towards such institutionalisation as has been recommended in research (Banken, 2001; 2003; Putters, 2005; Bekker, 2007; Morgan, 2008). Consideration must be made by the promoters and stakeholders in the HIA processes of the institutions ultimately to use the HIA, and without threatening the integrity of the process.

In terms of institutional working and the processes at play, partnership can be difficult and painstaking at times, as was identified with the Ballyfermot HIA. One respondent working within the health system stated that partnership working 'can be time consuming and difficult'.

One respondent who represented the local community on the steering group stated that there were clearly institutional constraints inhibiting the behaviour of certain individuals involved in the HIA process. However, these constraints, with regard to one key statutory body, were overcome once the relevant individuals became amenable to the HIA and the work being done, 'and they (the statutory bodies) listened and acted'.

Political dimension: do politics matter?

This study investigated the influence of a political dimension by asking the respondents to what extent did they believe politics at play between the varying interests in the conduct of the HIA. The responses to this question have been categorised into four groups. The existence of a political dimension at a micro-level (individuals) and macro-level (institutions) was identified, as well as the meaning of evidence and how that arose some tensions, and the nature and meaning of 'politics' during the HIA process. These themes are explored in the following section.

Individuals: the gatekeepers to the institutions

It was pointed out by an individual working within the health system that all individuals came to the HIA with their own agendas and interests, as is illustrated in the following quotation:

> Each person has their own agenda, it's real life! (One statutory body) was reluctant at beginning, but then were most enthusiastic; maybe they feared health at the table.

This individual made particular reference to the local authority and the members representing that body as being sceptical at the beginning of the HIA. This point of view was reiterated by an interviewee from the community also, but the statements were qualified by pointing out how such local authority members became more enthusiastic and less fearful and unsure of the HIA as time went on in the process. This finding supports the continuation of capacity-building in HIA and awareness-raising of the instrument and approach within and across all sectors, including statutory, voluntary and community bodies and groups, and also highlights the value of experiential learning with the HIA instrument.

There were varying degrees of involvement and activity in the HIA identified by a member of the Institute of Public Health, who believed that some individuals came to the table with different levels of commitment: '(There were) no conflicting interests but varying degrees of involvement. Some time was spent around roles to be fulfilled by members. People came to the table with different degrees of willingness.' These degrees of willingness on the part of individuals in the process impacted on the HIA and increased the workload for some around the table, thus causing tensions and the potential for conflict.

Institutions: the gate and the building

A member from URBAN II believed there was more tension with members from the health services, as illustrated in the following:

> We ... strongly pushed for the HIA, and we pushed the community participation element. Some (individuals from statutory bodies) weren't as used to the community being involved as (our) staff was.

This statement illuminates the problem that can arise with intersectoral working in policy issues. One health services representative stated how partnership between the different sectors and institutions was very difficult. A respondent interviewed from the Institute of Public Health also reiterated this when discussing value systems of individuals coming to the process, stating that it would be of help if all individuals in the process clarified the values of the institution that they were representing at the table, in order to prevent conflict or tension further on in the HIA process.

It was also highlighted in the interviews how the attitude of some individuals towards the HIA process, coming from certain statutory institutions, would be to 'leave it to gather dust on the shelf' (URBAN II representative). Indeed, a member of the local authority qualified this fear, by stating that if

HIAs were deemed unworkable with unrealistic recommendations attached to them, then there was the danger that such 'documents will gather dust on shelves and never be used'.

However, on a more positive note, a senior engineering official within the local authority on the HIA steering group stated that whilst there 'probably was tension, it (the HIA) was a good opportunity to explain policies to those with a health background, and the process was useful'. The interviewee noted how much cross-sectoral and cross-institutional learning can come from such intersectoral instruments and approaches of working in policy areas.

Politics? Not here!

The mentioning of the term 'politics' during the interviews in this case study raised a few eyebrows amongst some respondents. Although these respondents, as all did in interviews from all four HIA cases, admitted to the presence of conflicting views and tensions during the HIA, it was a 'politics with a small p' and of no great issue. An individual from the local authority stated 'I wouldn't call it politics, just different focuses; the (health services) focused on methodology and process, and the (local authority) on outcomes.'

However, no great conflict of opinions hindered the HIA process to any large degree and any issues that arose during the process were dealt with openly within the framework of the HIA. They were facilitated within the HIA, which has been devised to allow for such traits of intersectoral working.

The role of value judgements in the HIA process

The complexity of the policy process was pointed out by the HIA expert member of the steering group, reflecting on the process as being 'a logical decision making path … (which in reality) is not like that at all. There are many complexities in the pathways of policy-making that need to be considered, especially when assessing the use of HIA for policy'.

Another important and related issue is the question of the role that values, beliefs and assumptions play in the policy process. The role of these values has been the topic of research in IA literature, and is being used as an explanatory factor in this study; to assess the influence of value judgement in the use of HIAs. Since no matter how rational the policy process may appear to be, it is ingrained with value systems, beliefs and subjective irrationalism (Carley, 1980; Krnv and Thissen, 2000; Weston, 2002; Bekker *et al.*, 2004).

The following themes arose from the interviews. The varying ideas and opinions of the respondents in the role that values play, and the influence they may have in the policy process, arose from the interview data.

Community

Many responses regarding the existence and role of values pertained to the value placed on the opinion of the Ballyfermot community within the HIA process. Although the value placed on the community's perspective may be of little concern to policy-makers when they are formulating policy in years gone by, the new wave of consultative and bottom-up approaches to policy-making within local government and within the centralised HSE is given more attention and greater activity. This sentiment was emphasised in the interviews, from respondents of both community and statutory perspectives. Great value was placed on the views of the community during the HIA process, and this point was positively affirmed during the interview with a respondent from a community group who sat on the steering group (local resident of Ballyfermot and community representative on the HIA). The steering group informed the community of its recommendations, and feedback from the community was incorporated into the final HIA document. One issue that was amended was that greater attention was to be given to the elderly and disabled in the public transport system as pointed out by a member of the health services, which was then implemented on the ground with traffic and safety measures by the local authority, as confirmed in an interview with an official from DCC.

The Local Action Group (LAG) (known locally as the Impact Group) was set up in 2008 to implement the HIA recommendations specifically for the community to deliver. This group had difficulty sustaining itself once the HIA finished and once URBAN II input was reduced. For a time it was coordinated by the RAPID project coordinator until it dissolved due to lack of resources and an increasing workload. However, although the Impact Group did not sustain itself within the local community, it did have a direct influence on a number of local health initiatives in the area, such as the creation of the primary health care centre and the Cold Weather Response Initiative, as was confirmed by a member of DCC working in the Ballyfermot Area Office (phase II of the study).

Values

The response of those interviewed regarding the role of values and beliefs in the policy process, and thus in the role of the value placed on HIAs which may go on to influence policy, was a proposition widely accepted. One member of the Institute of Public Health developed the point further and reflected that it would be helpful if all stakeholders would clarify their value systems early on in the process, so as to establish the beliefs and attitudes people had of HIAs, informed policy-making and consultative policy aiding instruments and approaches such as IA frameworks. A member of URBAN II stated vehemently how 'values and attitudes of people involved were definitely there' and their role throughout the process of the HIA, and in the aftermath, was an important factor to consider when evaluating the use, or non-use, of the HIA knowledge and evidence.

Institutional complexity

One member of the local authority stated 'it is my belief that it's (HIA) good, but practicability and so many institutions involved is a problem'. The respondent discussed the role that many value systems played in the process, and how this complexity can complicate the development of the HIA instrument and approach in practice, and can inhibit its success and therefore usability, in the future.

Negative attitudes towards HIA

There were some negative opinions and attitudes expressed towards the HIA process. This may have had a role in the development of the process during the conduct of the assessment. It also may inhibit its use by the members, and their affiliated institutions, into the future, as the HIA report was being used on an ongoing basis, according to many of those interviewed. A member of the local authority stated 'I believe you need research for informed decisions but I found this a woolly exercise'. This individual went to say that the HIA was not geared towards achievable outcomes or deliverables, but instead was more concerned with the process being rigorous and methodical. Variants of this opinion were discussed in the interviews with the other members of the same institution. This respondent went to say that 'the process than (the) product was more important here'. Realistic HIA recommendations was a highlighted issue also in the evaluation of the Ballyfermot HIA (Kearns and Pursell, 2007). This negative perception and experience may be explained as a clash of institutional values. However, whatever the reasoning, these opinions of the HIA process may impact on these officials becoming involved in HIAs in the future.

Must be implementable

Following on from the above point, an associated issue related to the HIAs being realistic and providing achievable recommendations. If unachievable suggestions are made in the HIA, a negative impression is then formed of the process, which would impact negatively on it into the future. This may shape prejudices against the instrument and approach and inform attitudes, assumptions, values and beliefs that act as constraints in the area of HIA work further down the line.

One respondent working in the Ballyfermot area as a local authority official stated that it is the lacking deliverability of HIAs that can be a constraining factor, 'especially if someone had something completely off the wall. Going back to the point of what's realistic. It would be a disservice to HIA if not feasible recommendations are put into the report'.

A member of URBAN II reiterated this point of realism in recommendations in response to this interview question. This respondent went to say that the involvement of the Green Party in national politics at the time, and their consideration of informed policy-making as part of their party manifestos and principles, and in areas of environmental health and wellbeing, 'will influence what's incorporated into policy planning, so their influence might seep downwards'. The interviewee believed in the influence of national politics and the political ideologies on local activities, and in particular believed a political party and their value systems would impact on the development and use of HIAs in local policy-making circles. Governments in the new millennium have made similar calls for more participative policy-making, however there is no formal structure to facilitate such bottom-up participative approaches to national policy-making in the jurisdiction.

Need for legislation

A senior official of the local authority stated, in response to being asked about values, that the fact that HIAs are not enshrined in legislation makes it difficult to become incorporated into mainstream policy-making. Therefore it is difficult to break the mould of the values and attitudes that are associated with other IAs. For instance, he stated that HIA was, at times, perceived as 'piggy-backing on EIA', which he viewed as a negative phenomenon as it was associated with making EIA more cumbersome and difficult for officials. Such an attitude can thus impact negatively on the value placed upon HIAs as policy-aiding instruments and approaches.

Persuading institutions and people

Majone (1989) argues that the policy process can be manipulated and persuaded as to what is, and is not, feasible. According to this work, Majone proposes that policy arguments are founded on value judgements, and not always based on rational and logical thinking processes of policy-makers. This assertion is true in the case of the Ballyfermot HIA, as far as the interviewees were concerned. One interviewee working in the Ballyfermot area as a local authority official stated that 'people are open to persuasion, to be persuaded by the valid argument, and there were many views around the table'. He went on to say that if the HIA process fails to produce concrete and achievable deliverables, a disservice will be done to the instrument and approach. However, if solid and realistic recommendations are suggested, then those around the table, and outside the HIA process, could be persuaded of its benefit and its usefulness for policy-making.

Another member of the local authority also made the point that 'people have to sell the value of HIA and what it is', the benefits of the instrument and approach and the solidity of its outcomes. A further point associated with this was developed by a member of the health services who sat on the steering group, who reflected on the point of 'how communication is packaged' to those outside and inside the HIA group was important, so as to get as many supporters of the process on board as possible. The more people in support of the HIA, the greater the chance that it will be accepted and used by policy-makers. A certain amount of 'politicising of HIA' was involved, in order to spread the word and broadcast its practicability. At the end of the Ballyfermot HIA a big launch event was organised. The Lord Mayor at the time was a vocal locally elected representative of the area (at the time of HIA, he was a city councillor, and at the time of writing is representing the area in the national parliament), and he launched the report in DCC headquarters. Interviews were given at the event to a national broadcaster and the HIA was written about in the *Irish Times Health Supplement* (national broadsheet newspaper in the Republic of Ireland). The project also won the Irish Healthcare Awards 2005 for best innovation practice. Such activities further highlighted the work of the HIA, disseminated its findings, and portrayed to a wider audience the feasibility and usefulness of HIAs for policy-making.

Knowledge use for policy development

Each interviewee was asked to reflect on the extent that the HIA was used in policy processes. This section presents the responses to these reflections and discussions.

HIA recommendations

A member of the HIA steering group working within the health services stated that some recommendations were implemented, and admitted that some were not implemented. Kearns and Pursell (2007) conducted an evaluation of the Ballyfermot HIA and concluded that the recommendations that were not yet implemented were just not feasible or realistic. This is a lesson for future HIAs; to ensure recommendations are feasible and deliverable. It was raised also in the interviews for this study as was previously mentioned.

However, various local activities were implemented on the ground, which derived from the HIA and its recommendations for action. Examples of these were cited by some of the interviewees, for instance, the change of the sequencing of traffic lights near Tesco shopping centre; healthy eating and walking programmes were commenced as a result of the findings of the poor health status of the local community; an improvement of local mental health services was identified during data collection of the HIA; and a project promoting physical exercise was started, as well as a Health Fair held in the Tesco shopping centre. In addition, a local authority official stated that 'Dublin Bus (a statutory transport body in RoI) has taken (the recommendation) on board to make travel safer. Bus stops are now safer for the disabled'. However Dublin Bus was not represented on the steering group, which would have limited its capacity to adopt more recommendations and to contribute to the HIA.

Policy environment

A number of responses dealt with issues relating to the policy environment and how the HIA would influence it, both concurrently and into the future.

A member of the HIA steering group working with the health services stated that all city and county managers (of all local government authorities) in the country received a copy of the HIA report in 2005. This act was one which aimed at raising awareness of the health impacts of traffic and transport, of raising awareness of the HIA instrument and approach, and in providing evidence to such high-level local authority officials. Feedback from such individuals was deemed as 'positive' by this interviewee. However there is no evidence to suggest that this act of dissemination initiated others in local authorities to start HIA projects. In relation to the policy environment and the use of HIAs, the danger of the instrument and approach being viewed as an 'administrative burden' and used as a 'tick the box exercise' was highlighted. This manner of dealing with HIA in such a obligatory way is already being conducted with regard to other IAs in RoI and is a danger for HIA also.

Regarding the influence of the Ballyfermot HIA, one respondent from the Institute of Public Health reflected that it would inform policy in an incremental manner, as 'it may drip into policy, (although it would) not be an explosive contribution to policy but may inform it indirectly', and was good for the future. A senior official of the local authority also stated that the HIA has informed city council policy indirectly to inform local transport plans. This drip-feed idea of HIAs' indirect but tangible influence on policy development was raised also in phase II of the research, thus highlighting the slow but steady contribution HIA can make to policy-making.

A member of a community group stated that there was a lack of clear policy coordination between DCC and South County Dublin Council, as was seen by the lack of cross-information on traffic management and traffic lights sequencing. Ballyfermot is based on the border between the two local authorities. This apparent lack of policy coordination, which was however rebuked by a member of the local authority when questioned on it, does not bode well for policy-making processes at local government level that HIAs are aiming to influence and inform. The ongoing changes in the local government system at the time of writing may improve these coordination issues, or not. This remains to be seen.

Another interviewee working within the health services stated that for the future of HIAs, where people are coming from conceptually needs to be accounted for, especially when attempting to use such HIAs to influence policy. This individual also stated the importance of raising the awareness of this Ballyfermot HIA and of disseminating its findings, which happened by presenting at the sixth HIA International Conference (Birmingham, 2005), presenting at the Healthy Cities Network in Belfast, and by sharing the experience at the comprehensive training days, as organised by the IPH.

Political advocacy

When asked whether or not the HIA had been used in policy, one interviewee from URBAN II stated that locally elected councillors (of the local government authority) were made aware of it during a presentation made by a member of the steering group at a Local Area Committee meeting, and the HIA in turn made the elected representatives aware of the health implications of traffic and transport in the area. There is a potential for the HIA to be used in local electoral politics, as a political advocacy tool, according to one respondent from URBAN II. Whether or not HIA is designed for such advocacy is a topic of debate within the HIA community and was discussed in Chapter 2.

Sustainability of the HIA

One member of the health services stated that the LAG (known locally as the Impact Group) had been 'very effective, facilitated previously by URBAN II and now to be facilitated by DCC, which is a positive move'. As phase II of the study showed, the group dissolved subsequently. However the group and the findings of the HIAs informed and influenced a number of health related initiatives in the area, such as the creation of the primary health care centre and the Cold Weather Response Initiative.

Part III: update on the Traffic and Transport HIA

In 2014 interviews were conducted as part of phase II of the study with two members of the Ballyfermot HIA steering group, as well as exploratory discussions with members of the community, DCC and the public health services. At this stage, nine years after the HIA was conducted, many people who sat on the steering group, and who were interviewed in 2007 and 2008, had left their positions. A number of follow-up assessments of the HIA have been conducted, the first being the assessment of effectiveness of the HIA (Lavin and Metcalfe, 2007a) and then the official evaluation of the HIA (Kearns and Pursell, 2007). An assessment of the impacts of the HIA on intersectoral partnerships in local policy-making and on community participation was also carried out (Pursell and Kearns, 2012). The latter study included interviews with twenty-one key respondents involved in the HIA and from within the community and local organisations. The study illustrated similar positive impacts of the HIA as was found during its examination in this chapter, including a facilitation of community learning through the work of the LAG and an increase in awareness and understanding of the determinants of health. Pursell and Kearns (2012) found that there were differing views on HIA's role, with the community viewing it more as an advocacy tool, and service providers saw it more as a way to enable greater networking and collaboration. This tension exists within HIA development and is a topic under constant debate in public health circles, as discussed in Chapter 2. Although the Ballyfermot HIA did result in improved and increased community participation in local affairs, additional training and space for reflection for service providers and policy-makers would be useful prior to an HIA being conducted, so as to rectify in some way the power imbalances between the sectors (Pursell and Kearns, 2012), thus informing policies in an all-inclusive manner. In terms of longer term policy outcomes, the fact that the HIA was retrospective limited its ability to inform the policy process (Lavin and Metcalfe, 2007a), and some of the initiatives referred to in the recommendations of the HIA would have occurred in the absence of the HIA, which makes it difficult to directly assess the impact of the HIA on the policy process (Kearns and Pursell, 2007). Also the fact that the local authority and local health service providers were not obliged or required to implement all recommendations to the letter, meant that the full impact of the HIA on longer term policy development was always going to be limited. This point echoes the sentiment that was raised in Chapter 3, that HIA without a legislative basis or not being part of an official business plan of an organisation means that the chances of it being fully adopted and used within policy-making circles are very limited. Also much transport policy is decided and planned at the national level, which makes the degree to which an HIA can impact on local decision-making procedures in order to inform policies challenging (Kearns and Pursell, 2007). This is an issue connected with the ever decreasing powers and functions at local government level, with more powers and directives coming from the national government. In a discussion, a respondent from DCC working in the area on social and community affairs stated that although once URBAN II ceased to exist in the area and the impetus for the HIA Impact Group faded away, the HIA did continue to have a concrete impact on the local area, as illustrated in the following:

> I tried to keep it going but the workload was too much at the time. But although the group ceased to exist, a number of initiatives in the area came about as a direct result of the HIA. Such as the HIA being the forerunner of initiatives, for example the Primary Care Health Centre, environmental

improvement that was taken up by the Parks Department and Community and Social Development Department in DCC, and also the Cold Weather Response Initiative.

This demonstrates that the HIA continues to this day, has influenced health-related activities in the area, and is still considered as a key action and source of evidence by the local authority.

HIA on the Draft Air Quality Action Plan, 2006 (Belfast, Northern Ireland)

Part I: description

BCC elected for an HIA to be conducted on the Draft Air Quality Action Plan in 2005 (Belfast City Council, 2006). Belfast Healthy Cities, which has pioneered the use of HIA, supported the council and led the steering group when carrying out this comprehensive prospective HIA. Rapid appraisal and community workshops were conducted in the designated Air Quality Management Areas (AQMAs) in Belfast city (Institute of Public Health, 2007). The Air Quality Action Plan and the HIA report were launched at the same event in May 2006 in BCC.

BCC has a statutory responsibility to develop an action plan to improve the air quality of the city. The council opted for the use of HIA, alongside the drafting of the plan, as it was an approach which provided 'an opportunity for stakeholders to make suggestions that will minimise any negative aspects and also improve the way in which plans are implemented' (Belfast City Council, 2006: 81). The HIA was funded by the Environment and Heritage section of the Department of the Environment and BCC. This HIA can be categorised as a comprehensive, prospective one since the draft plan was already quite far advanced in its formulation stage, and would not be categorised as a concurrent HIA process. Lavin and Metcalfe (2007b) also propose this assertion. The National Air Quality Strategy, which was first published in 1997 and a subsequent nationwide UK strategy produced in 2000, indicates what is expected from local authorities in order to improve air quality in their areas. The overarching premise of this strategy is that clean air is essential for the health of the population.

In 2004 the council conducted a review of air quality in the city, measuring eight health-based pollutants. The result was that four AQMAs were formed. These areas are ones which are expected to exceed the pollutant target levels for nitrogen dioxide and particulate matter (PM10), as laid out in the National Air Quality Strategy. The areas are located along busy arterial routes (Ison, 2006).

The rationale for the completion of this HIA was to ensure that successful and achievable solutions to air quality problems were proposed by the local authority. It was discovered that during the implementation of air quality action plans in local authorities in England (in accordance with the National Strategy), numerous proposals, as set forth in the action plans, had negative knock-on effects on an adjacent area and community. The HIA process is a structured framework for the consideration of all possible intended and unintended consequences of policy (Kemm and Parry, 2004), and would be beneficial for the formulation of the Belfast Draft Air Quality Action Plan. The HIA was envisaged to mitigate the problems of unintended knock-on effects as experienced in parts of England. The council's environmental health manager has stated also that 'as statutory agencies we have an ethical and social duty to ensure the measures that are proposed are tested to some degree with the population on which they will have an effect' (Toland, 2006: 3). It was the goal of the HIA to ensure the health gains in the action plan would be maximised, and negative impacts would be minimised, as far as practicable.

It was discovered during an interview with an official working in the local authority involved in the HIA that the idea of conducting an HIA came from attending an air quality conference in England. This individual was moved by evidence presented on the linkages between the physical environment and health and wellbeing, and came to believe that carrying out an HIA would improve the air quality action plan.

Specific objectives were not outlined in the report of the HIA (Ison, 2006). However, consultation workshops that were held with relevant stakeholders were centred on the main themes of the Draft Air Quality report, as are indicated in the following:

1. Initiatives to promote walking and cycling in Belfast.
2. Initiatives to promote increased use of transport in Belfast.
3. Initiatives to promote improved vehicle fleet management.
4. Initiatives to encourage the uptake of greener energy options by large organisations.
5. Implementation of policies that will contribute to reducing air pollution.
6. Highway and road improvements that will contribute to reducing air pollution.
7. Marketing and education initiatives to raise awareness among the public. (Ison, 2006: 11)

During the four workshops that were held in the summer of 2005, different stakeholders were consulted on varying aspects of the abovementioned seven themes, as will be outlined in the HIA methodology section below.

Stakeholder involvement

Stakeholders involved in the HIA were drawn from the public, private, voluntary and community sectors. Residents from two of the AQMAs (the M1/Westlink and the Ormeau Road communities), were involved in the HIA consultation workshops. Workshops were also held at two schools which are in, or close to, two of the AQMAs (Strandtown Primary School and St. Malachy's Primary School). A number of those interviewed in this study were involved in the HIA and also in the formulation of the Air Quality Action Plan.

Although an HIA expert consultant was hired to lead the process, a steering group was established to oversee the management and completion of the HIA. There were thirty-five members in this group. A management team was also set up, which was a guiding force leading the steering group; this group consisted of six members drawn from BCC, Belfast Healthy Cities (BHC), the Department of Public Health and Nursing (health services) and the HIA expert consultant. In this Belfast HIA, eight people were included for interviews, all of which except one were conducted with management team or steering group members. An additional exploratory interview was carried out with an official working in the OFMDFM, in Castle buildings, Stormont, Belfast. This individual reflected on the IIA tool across government ministries, which is now known as Policy Toolkit. The Toolkit is informed by HIA and other IA frameworks (O'Mullane, 2008). Four people were interviewed in 2014 as part of phase II.

Belfast City Council

The Environmental Health section of the council, under the auspices of the Environmental Protection domain, was the driver of the HIA process from within that local authority. Three members sat on the management team. The leading individual from within BCC was the Environmental Health Manager in the council and was in this position at the time of the HIA. This individual was integral to the process, as without a high-level position of power and influence within the council administration, and the enthusiasm to commence the HIA, it would not have started. This individual was vital to the HIA. In addition, another member of the Environmental Health section of the council was involved in the HIA, on the management team.

Belfast Healthy Cities

Established in 1988, Belfast Healthy Cities (BHC) is the oldest partnership in the city. It plays a major role in promoting health partnerships and projects and is one of the first organisations to carry out HIAs in Belfast. It is one of the leading cities within the WHO European Healthy Cities Network. The organisation views its role as one to promote health on the political and social agenda, and included in this is an awareness and endorsement of the healthy urban planning approach. BHC plays a key role in promoting HIA as an important instrument and approach to ensure healthier urban planning in the formation of urban design and local area plans and city masterplans (Belfast Healthy Cities, 2007a; 2007b), and in the advancement of the HiAP agenda.

Expert HIA practitioner

The role of the HIA practitioner is one which is commonplace on such projects. There generally tends to be an experienced and dedicated practitioner and researcher who will conduct and lead the HIA, with the direction and support of a steering committee. In the study on the assessment of effectiveness of this HIA to support decision-making, Lavin and Metcalfe (2007b) found that the inclusion of the external consultant introduced more objectivity into the process which was a positive development for the HIA overall.

Department of Public Health and Nursing within the Eastern Health and Social Services Board (EHSSB) (this board has been restructured within the Public Health Authority)

This body was represented on the management team. The rationale underlying the inclusion of a dedicated public health specialist was to ensure matters relating to population health and the determinants of health were the sole focus and concern of one team member. This was to guarantee and guard the primary focus as one of health and wellbeing. The decision to include a representative from a public health background in the team was explained by a local authority official, who stated that 'we decided to get a health expert in it ... so it was a case of learning by doing at the beginning'.

Department of Regional Development (DRD), Roads Service

The Regional Transportation Strategy (RTS) for Northern Ireland, 2002 to 2012, was endorsed by the Northern Assembly in 2002. It identified the transportation agenda and funding allocation priorities until 2012. The DRD Roads Service's contributions to the Action Plan are based on the Belfast Metropolitan Transport Plan (BMTP), which completes in 2015. It ensures the strategic vision of the RTS is operationalised on the ground. The DRD Roads Service is a central government agency that works closely with local authorities.

Community groups

Community consultation workshops with residents of two of the AQMAs (M1/Westlink and the Ormeau Road communities), with two schools (Strandtown Primary School and St. Malachy's Primary School) and with individuals of the community, private and public sectors, were carried out as part of the HIA. Schools were inspired by the HIA and initiated health promoting campaigns and clean air programmes, including tree-planting areas on school grounds.

Institute of Public Health (IPH)
The Institute of Public Health is an all-island agency, which is based in Dublin and Belfast. It aims to address the island's public health needs by conducting research and informing governing departments of health requirements for the population. The Institute was represented in this HIA (on the steering group/management team).

HIA methodology

A literature review was conducted regarding other HIAs conducted on similar proposals elsewhere and data of the local area was used to establish a profile of the community. Workshops were held, during which time people were called upon to 'judge the effects of the draft Air Quality Action Plan on the health and wellbeing of people living and working in Belfast' (Ison, 2006: 13). One workshop was held for members of the public, private, voluntary and community sectors; workshops were held in two resident areas and in two local primary schools (Ison, 2006: 13).

HIA outcomes

Suggestions (which were specifically not termed as recommendations, as is the protocol of Ison) were established as a result of the stakeholder workshops. These suggestions were framed within the context of either reducing potential negative effects or enhancing potential positive effects of various air quality improvement initiatives. Suggestions were made by all stakeholders in relation to each of these seven areas. The Air Quality Action Plan, which was published in 2006, utilised evidence from each of the themed areas in the final report (Belfast City Council, 2006).

Policy process for the Draft Air Quality Action Plan for Belfast

The main institution using the evidence and knowledge from the HIA was BCC. This organisation was both the initiator of the process and the envisaged end user of the HIA for council policy. However, this local authority does not have any operational function over transport policy. In reality, this means that although the council can coordinate action on air quality, it has no statutory power to enforce the measures. This continues to be the case, as confirmed in an interview in 2014 by officials working in the local authority.

There is a direct relationship between the HIA on the draft plan (conducted in 2005; reported in 2006) and the outcome final plan (2006). Sparse information is available on the use of the evidence of the other key statutory, voluntary or community bodies (Belfast City Council, 2006). This was explored during the conduct of expert interviews with members of the management team (5), steering group (2), and others (3). Unlike the Ballyfermot HIA, no official evaluation of this HIA was conducted.

Part II: analysis

As with the other HIAs included in this study, interviews were carried out with respondents for this HIA case, which were in turn analysed. The results of this analysis are presented in the following section. The conceptual lens, as outlined in Chapter 2, provides the framework for the findings from the interview data. As stated already, in this Belfast HIA case study, a total of eight people were interviewed as part of phase I of the study (2007/8) and four in 2014 (phase II).

'Institutions matter': New Institutional Theory

A number of questions were asked during the interview phase of data collection, in order to establish the degree of influence the norms of institutions had over the use of the HIA report, and the knowledge that came from that and its preceding process.

Are institutions ready? The timing of HIA as a policy support instrument and approach

The timing of HIA as a policy support instrument and approach was asked during the interviews with steering group and management team members, so as to establish the perspective of those on the HIA steering group, which included decision-makers and representatives of statutory bodies.

Except for two respondents, all those who were interviewed stated that yes, the time was right and had come for HIAs to be used in policy-making.

The two respondents who did not agree on the timing of the HIA were more cautious in their appraisal of the HIA instrument and approach, stating that maybe the time had come to use HIAs in policy-making, but not stating an affirmative 'yes'. One of these individuals was from the DRD, and had a more reserved opinion of the HIA conducted on the action plan. This individual believed that the fact the HIA and action plan were conducted concurrently was unhelpful for the Air Quality Plan, as outlined in the following quotation: 'There's an issue about how it influences the action plan, they were done together and there's a problem with timing … they were done in parallel and (it was) like ticking boxes.' An individual from another statutory body who was involved in the HIA also was more cautious in evaluating the timeliness and appropriateness of the instrument and approach.

Five of those interviewed stated that yes, based on their experience with the Belfast City Air Quality Plan (Belfast City Council, 2006), the time had come to use HIAs in public policy. These respondents worked in the statutory and voluntary sectors. A representative from the health services stated that it was a 'workable instrument and approach and we should be using it', and there is a need to raise its profile by using HIA. A member of BHC agreed that the time was right to use evidence from HIA but believed that the ongoing political and administrative reform could hinder the process of use and integration of HIA. One local authority official believed the time was right for the use of HIAs in policy, qualifying her statement with 'was there ever a right time? It was never going to be an easy task so we just decided to get on with it and see what happens. [Members of the HIA steering committees] felt it was the right time and a way to get it [HIA approach] in the back door to influence strategic agendas'. This highlights again the experiential learning aspect when conducting HIAs for the first time; a learning-by-doing approach was acknowledged with the HIA. A member of the Institute of Public Health concurred that the time had come to use HIAs, as 'there's a need for evidence in policy, especially looking at health in all polices. Evidence shows to date if you don't have evidence then nothing is going to change'.

Further to whether or not the timing was right for HIAs, the interviewees went on to expand on their responses to this question. Several factors came from the interviews such as the institutional factors which were present in enabling and hindering the use of HIAs. The policy process was cited as a factor in the timeliness of the instrument and approach. The public administration reform programme ongoing in Northern Ireland (in 2007 and 2008, and also at the time of writing in 2014) was found to impact on the use and acceptance of HIAs. The nature of community engagement, the IIA, and the spirit of HIA, the meaning of health (conceptualisation of health) and the lack of statutory recognition surfaced also as factors affecting the opinions on timeliness and suitability of HIA as a policy-aiding instrument and approach in the current day phenomenon of policy-making.

First, a number of issues relating to the impact of institutional forces upon the use and acceptance of HIA arose during the interviews. One member of BHC stated that there was commitment from the NIHE and BCC to mainstream HIA for all projects, programmes and policies. There were also ongoing constructive discussions with the OFMDFM regarding the formal establishment of IIA, which would incorporate the consideration of health impacts with statutory recognition in the long run.

Leadership within the institutional organisations was identified as a necessary ingredient for HIAs to be conducted smoothly, and for their evidence to be used in public policy thereafter. This point was raised by a member of BHC who believed that the time had come to use evidence from HIAs in policy, as long as top-level leadership was in support of the concept, which was overall the case in the Belfast Air Quality HIA.

One interviewee working in the local authority explained the institutional difficulties in formulating the Air Quality Action Plan. Getting the various statutory bodies who work in the policy sectors of transport, roads, housing and urban development on board was identified as challenging. The reality of the situation was that the delivery of the Air Quality Action Plan is a statutory requirement and priority for the council, but was not for the other bodies required to participate in the HIA. The respondent said this was 'hugely frustrating, it took us nearly two years to get the plan together … and planning (the statutory planning services) never came to table, and that was a huge partner not there before the HIA started'. Many of the key stakeholders were central government departments and were not accustomed to inter-relating their agendas with others; 'central government departments work alone unlike local government, and it's very, very difficult to influence their agendas'. Hopefully when the Community Planning clause of the Local Government Act (Northern Ireland) 2014 is implemented, there will be greater involvement of the planning services in endeavours such as HIA. The reform of local government will also involve a transferring of some of the planning services to the local authorities, which should also benefit instruments and approaches, such as HIA, towards building healthier public policies, as mentioned by local authority officials in an interview in phase II of the study.

Challenges in doing the HIA on the Air Quality Action Plan were identified by respondents. The difficulty stemmed from individuals using different sources for their evidence of air quality, with one sourced locally and the other from the London Health Observatory. However, although this instance demonstrated some reluctance of the upper echelons of knowledge and power to accept evidence which incorporates outside research and academic evidence, overall the local authority willingly accepted the evidence that came from the HIA.

A point raised in the interviews was that there was a problem with cooperation and mutual sharing of information across institutional boundaries; 'in broader terms people are very self-focused and don't inter-relate with other people's agendas'. A member of BHC reflected a major issue of some 'huge partners not (being) there, even before we did the HIA'. Two of these major partners were the planning services and roads service. The latter did come to the table during the HIA process but the former group never did. The HIA could not achieve maximum benefit from the process when the planning services, a vital partner, are missing.

Second, the policy process arose as a factor impacting upon the use of HIAs. A member working in the DRD believed that the issue was 'the timing in the policy process', that the conducting of the HIA and draft action plan concurrently was problematic for the HIA. A representative from the local authority believed that the fact that this was the first HIA being conducted was detrimental to the instrument and approach, as at times it made a less than positive impression on policy-makers.

A member of the IPH stated that 'evidence was needed for policy', which was why HIA's time had come as there was increasing evidence needed for informed policy-making. An official working in the local authority also believed that evidence coming from the process was important, as well as health's place on policy-makers' agendas.

Third, the issue of public administration reform arose as a major factor regarding the timeliness of HIAs, and the manner in which the instrument could succeed in the current institutional climate of public administrative reform. The reinstitution of central power in Stormont in 2006/7 and the political and administrative changes of the RPA have influenced the conduct and use of HIAs. This was reaffirmed during the interviews conducted in 2014. A member of BHC felt the opportunity for the institutionalisation of HIAs during this time of change was not seized, which was reaffirmed also in an interview in 2014. A member of the local authority stated that circa 2005 and 2006 there was tension across all statutory bodies regarding what the RPA would bring, and this proved a major influence in the level of engagement of statutory bodies in the HIA: 'In theory (it is) a good tool for collaboration but the timing, the RPA was a big influence, was started to be muted, (some statutory bodies) were nervous that they'd come under local government and the planning service.' This individual believed that because of the increased uncertainty arising from the RPA process, it would be more difficult to conduct the HIA. Overall, it was a case of 'now or never' regarding the conduct of this HIA on the Draft Air Quality Action Plan in the institutional climate at the time.

Fourth, the 'the proposers didn't have a problem with what came from the community groups, and that fed into the action plan, they took that on board alright, they were positive and would say it did influence the action plan'. A positive aspect of HIAs in relation to the evidence derived from the process, is that all stakeholders involved in the process are, in the end, in possession of evidence that they can use at a later date and in other proposals or in lobbying policy-makers on other issues. This was the situation with the other HIAs explored in this book.

Fifth, there is a case to be made for the development of an IIA, which would incorporate the main tenets of all IAs inhabiting the policy process at the moment, as pointed out by a member of BHC. This has been developed to form the now instated Policy Toolkit in the Belfast Assembly (devolved parliament).

The sixth category that arose from the interviews was the nature of HIA and the manner in which the instrument and approach was shaped in order to ensure it was appropriate for use in current policy. It became clear during the interviews, which was not apparent from reading the documentary evidence alone, that one of the primary reasons behind conducting the HIA was to broker cooperation between the stakeholders in the action plan. It was carried out in order to try 'to influence them (leading agencies involved in the formation of the action plan), influencing them with another new tactic … and I thought, why not give it a go and let these (people) have a think about the wider determinants of health and what the implications of (transport) structures might be'. HIA is often used for this purpose (as a brokering device), however it is not often explicitly stated with those participating in the process. If an HIA is conducted for this reason, then expectations of the process to produce easier intersectoral relations need to be realistic and not overly hopeful. HIA cannot, and is not designed to, meet every hope and expectation.

The seventh category that came from the interviews in response to the timing of HIAs was the conceptualisation of health, and how it impacted on the progress of the approach. A member of BHC stated that there were challenges during the conduct of the project with the various non-health sector stakeholders around the meaning of health. This individual also explained there were difficulties with those from a public health background as their understanding of health was from a biomedical health perspective. A member of the local authority felt that doing the HIA was a good way to inform statutory professionals of the wider determinants of health, which was raised again by members of the local authority during the interviews conducted in 2014, as a long-term benefit of conducting the HIA.

The final category was the lack of statutory recognition of HIA, which hindered the overall development of HIAs in Northern Ireland, as raised by a member of BHC. Although it was clear in many respects that the timing was appropriate for the use of HIAs in policy, there were a number of factors influencing this use, as have been outlined in this section.

Normative dimension: do institutions shape behaviour?

The use of institutional theory in this study was to establish the extent of the influence that certain institutions have on the use of HIAs and the knowledge that came from them, which was intended to inform policy.

Those interviewed in this case were stakeholders in the HIA process. They were on the management team and steering group as representatives of their relevant bodies, be it from statutory institutions of the local government and health sector and voluntary bodies. The steering group was made up of an eclectic range of statutory bodies, all having an interest professionally in the Air Quality Action Plan. First, at institutional, HIA process and policy process levels, a number of constraining factors upon behaviour were elicited, such as a number of key stakeholders were missing from the process, or not engaged fully, and some of the players that were involved were not accustomed to sharing information or perspectives across institutional boundaries. The ability of leading statutory bodies involved in the HIA to influence other institutions and their policy agendas was difficult, bordering on impossible, since there was no legislative or statutory requirement for other institutions and bodies to take on board the findings of the HIA. That the HIA process was a new concept, and that it is not compulsory/mandatorily required, were identified as constraining factors within the institutional context. Within the policy process, institutional constraints were identified regarding the use and acceptance of the HIA. According to one member of the health services there were constraints 'because of the timing of the action plan'. In this individual's opinion, conducting the action plan and the HIA concurrently made their completion within their respective time frames very difficult. A member of the local authority stated that the 'policy process is not static, there is no guarantee the HIA will be used'. The uncertain and quick-moving nature of the policy process is a constraining factor upon the use of HIAs and the findings of the process.

Second, gathering local evidence and the way it is collected was deemed a constraint for the HIA approach. The way that evidence was collected in the local area to provide the evidence base for the HIA, which would in turn hope to influence and inform the policy process, was regarded as constraining. Different bodies collected evidence differently, and were not keen or willing to share information across institutional boundaries. The lack of evidence for policy was constraining, which was identified, in turn, as the main rationale behind conducting the HIA – to fill the evidence gap. These points were raised by respondents working in BHC and in the local authority.

Third, community human resources played a constraining role in this case study, as there was little community infrastructure around the issue of physical development in the four AQMAs. It was a constraint on the process that there was not already in existence a strong community spirit, which could work with and on the HIA.

Political dimension: do politics matter?

This study looked at the influence of a political dimension; by asking the interviewees to what extent did they believe that politics were at play between the varying interests in the conduct of the HIA. The responses to this question have been categorised into three groups. The political dimension at a micro-level (individuals) and macro-level (institutions) was identified. The use of

HIA as an advocacy instrument and approach was highlighted also, as well as expectations of the process as identified by respondents in the study.

Individuals: the gatekeepers to the institutions
With regards to politics at play, both in the conduct and aftermath of the HIA, some of the interviewee responses related to the fact that perhaps some individuals on the steering group were not fully committed to the idea of the HIA, and were defending their institutional line while involved in the process. Interviewees referred to cross-institutional politics. This latter point was more apparent on the steering group, as those on the management team were more united and collaborative than the former group; 'everyone was backing their organisations and were defending their own areas. For instance, representatives from [some statutory bodies] were not going to say anything that would result in them having to dramatically change their policy or plans'. This point was reiterated by a local authority respondent, who stated that while 'there was softening, people came to the table with [their] organisation's perspective'. Indeed, however tense or implicitly political the interactions were between the key stakeholders, a 'key outcome is building professional relationships with people, especially good people'. That is to say, that this respondent as a member of the management team found that there were some key bright, innovative thinkers across the organisations that were involved in the HIA, and believed that meeting and collaborating with such policy entrepreneurs was an important outcome from the process. On the other side, there were individuals who were unreceptive to the HIA, to the findings and the essence of collaborative working which is part of the spirit of HIA. However during the process of the HIA, as was also the case in the Ballyfermot HIA with statutory members, some members can become supporters of the process once they acknowledge the benefits of such working, as illustrated in the following quotation: 'one department who came along and were very "closed book" about it all and had made up their mind beforehand, but then after some group meetings and after doing up the suggestions he was very much in support of the HIA, so that's a "win"' (local authority respondent).

Institutions: the gate and the building
One respondent from the health services stated that there were very little politics at play during the conduct of the HIA, apart from 'politics with a small p, as it was a multi sectoral and multi disciplinary process' with many stakeholders involved. Other interviewees were more convinced that there were institutional politics at play, across the institutional boundaries involved; 'there were a lot of politics, but not very overt. I wouldn't understand the politics between them (statutory bodies from the sectors of health, transport and regional development)', stated a member of BHC.

On the other side, there were tensions between central government departments and the local authority, as stated by the respondent from the DRD: 'there's always tensions in terms of departments (central government), seen as directorial, and then local councils, and it seems to me that local councils always want more power.' This point about working not only across sectors but also across tiers of government and governance is an important one to acknowledge in partnership working and inter-agency negotiations.

The NIHE was identified as an exceptional body, which was 'really a forward thinking agency; it's unlike other departments and agencies, where it's just like pulling teeth' (respondent from BHC).

A member of BHC continued with this sentiment:

> The housing executive (NIHE) is the only one really driving it (HIA) on, but that's the nature of the organisation; always up for change, they're sharp, on the ball, up to date, working at a local level with very difficult communities. And they see HIA as a very positive tool which helps too.

It was obvious based on informal conversations with other individuals involved in the Belfast HIA that the NIHE has an excellent reputation as an innovative organisation in NI. Where the institutional make-up in this HIA is concerned, the NIHE is ahead of all others in terms of innovation and flexibility, and is willing to allow others to enter the metaphorical institutional gate and building with more openness and willingness than other institutions. Although to this day HIA is not a statutory obligation of NIHE, the way the organisation works means it is already adopting a health lens to its policies and practices, and its ways of working are conducive to the ethos and spirit of HIA.

HIA: an advocacy tool?

The respondent from the DRD explained an opinion that the HIA may have been used as a tool for the local authority to endorse its view on the issue of transport and roads, since the local authority is keen to reduce the number of roads built, which contradicts the policy of the DRD. The following quotation illustrates the view that the HIA instrument and approach was perceived to advocate one particular viewpoint; that of the leaders and primary users of the HIA:

> At one stage there were tensions between how we're regurgitating what's in (the) transport plan and the HIA and draft plan, for instance we want to put in certain roads and there's great tension because the council doesn't want certain roads, would this HIA be seen as endorsing their view? There was a lot of playing around with words.

The extent to which HIA can be used as an implicit political means to a political end is an issue that was pertinently raised by this interviewee.

What do we expect from HIA?

One respondent from BHC raised the question of expectations around HIA, and that they need to be clarified when commencing a process. There are a number of priorities that the HIA tool can work towards, such as 'placing it (health) on someone's agenda, engaging communities, engaging stakeholders'. However, as raised by this individual, it is not a one-size-fits-all process, and what is expected from the process should be communicated and elucidated at the beginning, which to a large extent was not done in the HIA on the Air Quality Draft Action Plan.

The role of value judgements in the HIA process

The role that values, beliefs and assumptions play in the policy development process was highlighted during the study. Often such values are implicit and underlying behaviours and actions, unbeknown to people involved in policy development processes of every kind. Interviews with respondents from the Belfast case revealed a number of issues, such as values of institutions and organisations, impact of values in the policy process, values around health, valuing the contributions to the HIA process and the role of HIA champions in organisations.

Institutional and organisational values

In response to this question about values and decisions made based on value judgements, the interviewees were confident that values, and value judgements regarding the use of HIA evidence, played a role.

A respondent from the local authority illustrated this by saying:

> There were constraints in having so many organisations involved, so many agendas and budget pressures to consider and the HIA was looking at things in isolation but within each organisation it wasn't going to be acted through in isolation; it needs to be looked at within the entire organisational plan.

Another respondent from the local authority explained how it was 'difficult to make strategic changes with the big guys, values are not the same across institutions'. It was difficult, according to this individual, to implement change and ensure the use of the HIA across the stakeholder institutions involved in the Draft Action Plan, due to the varying value systems in each of the institutions. For instance, sectors working closely on transport and planning service issues were identified as reticent, whilst the NIHE have organisational values which welcome such an instrument as HIA.

Indeed, the values of the city council are service-focused, although this orientation is changing but will take time, as a respondent from the local authority reflected in the following:

> The values of (the local authority) is very service focused, service delivery focused and also the health aspect is very integral to that, improving the quality

> of life for future generations is a corporate mission and it's changed slightly in the last year, we've moved towards value creation maps but I'll not bore you with them, but it's to improve health, and quality of health is a major aspect as well as customer orientation.

This change in corporate mission is a part of the reform agenda for local government, in reorienting local authorities to prioritise broader issues around social, economic, health and environmental wellbeing as well as continuing to be service-provision focused.

The lack of statutory recognition of HIA also implied a value judgement from an institutional and central government policy level; without accordance of legislative footing of HIAs, the credibility of the instrument and approach will be doubted by statutory players involved in the city council's policy-making environment, as raised by a respondent from the local authority.

Values in policy process

A respondent from the health services reflected on her view that 'values played a positive role in the policy process', and especially in the promotion of the HIA on policy-makers' agendas, in relation to values conducive to knowledge generated from policy-informing instruments such as HIA. Also, according to a respondent from the DRD, 'you can't separate personal and professional values' and in this respondent's opinion this was the case in the perception of policy-makers of the HIA tool and the evidence arising from the process.

Valuing health

A respondent from BHC believed that 'the biggest challenge here is the economic versus health, wealth versus health' agenda. This issue is still fundamental to prioritising health at an institutional level. In interviews conducted in 2014, there appeared to be a growing awareness and recognition of the determinants of health and in adopting a HiAP approach in policy development within the local authority and with elected members of the city council. This bodes well for the consideration of health impacts of policy decisions into the future. However it is vital that all local authorities promote a HiAP approach across all activities, so that understanding of a holistic understanding of health and wellbeing is common knowledge across all units within the institution.

Valuing contributions to the HIA

The contributions to the HIA from the community stakeholders were vital to the process and valued by the statutory bodies. They were a most welcome aspect to the process as 'people aren't usually asked about their opinions for policy' as pointed out by the respondent from the Institute of Public Health.

It depends on the person ...
It was identified during the interviews that the influence of certain enthusiastic and innovative individuals can determine the successful implementation and use of an HIA in policy. Respondents from the local authority believed that 'it depends on who's the chief executive in the [local authority], depends on the leader. Because that filters right down through to all staff'. Apart from forward-thinking institutional leadership, certain individuals within organisations can make a difference too, and their absence is also a hindrance to the process: 'It's individual-dependent, yeah we'd formally ask them for individuals to come on board, and getting them was difficult in the beginning.' Institutional leadership for HIA is an important and necessary factor in the overall debate around institutionalising HIA and HiAP approaches, and this was highlighted within the Belfast HIA study.

Knowledge use for policy development

Respondents were asked about their opinions as to what extent the HIA was used in policy development and how useful the HIA was for the policy process. They were asked about how the knowledge generated from the HIA informed policy development, with the influences on knowledge use (as identified in the previous sections) in mind.

Action plan
According to a respondent from the health services, the HIA 'was useful and changes were made to the action plan'. This was reiterated by respondents from within the local authority, who also agreed that the suggestions from the HIA were taken on board into the action plan. The action plan's incorporation of the HIA's recommendations has been confirmed during the interviews with the stakeholders involved in the process from within the institution that formulated the action plan, namely the local authority.

However, a respondent from the local authority believed it was a mistake not to form an implementation group to follow-up, ensure and record that the suggestions from the HIA were fully implemented and taken on board:

> I think one of the limitations on our part was that we didn't establish an implementation group in it, having invested so much energy in it, so it's a lesson for us. And we've raised it at the air quality forum to ensure it is being used.

Ensuring sufficient implementation of HIA suggestions or recommendations is vital, as this respondent succinctly highlighted.

A respondent from the DRD believed that there was 'a flaw in the timing, the HIA being in parallel with the action plan'. From this individual's perspective, if the HIA had been conducted more in advance of the action plan, it would have had more impact.

Suggestions (HIA recommendations)
A respondent from the local authority, who was closest to the institutional machinery destined to use the HIA, and with the most knowledge of the process of HIA utilisation, admitted that while most suggestions from the HIA were incorporated, not all were fully implemented. However, a difficulty that was acknowledged by this individual was that other organisations had responsibility to implement HIA suggestions and it is difficult to ensure they are taken on board, as there is no statutory obligation for the suggestions to be implemented. This again highlights the necessity of a legislative basis for such approaches and endeavours.

Policy-making process (incidental benefits)
The rationale of the HIA was to inform the Air Quality Action Plan. However, it has been used for other purposes in policy; a number of incidental benefits to the HIA have been realised.

It was useful for developing a transport plan for the city council. A local authority respondent explained that 'the council is starting talks on developing a transport policy, even though we've no responsibility or powers in that area, we still need (to have) an opinion, a council line on the issue'. It also informed the council's submission for the planning services metropolitan area plan review, and more particularly used in the council concern over a fly-over, as illustrated in the following:

> A suggestion for a strategic road ... putting in a fly-over, linking south and east Belfast, might cause community severance and we articulated that by drawing from this HIA how communities are cut off, one half from another, because of such developments and what they think about it.

The HIA, although it was designed and formulated primarily to feed into the Air Quality Action Plan, will also be used to inform other city council plans and policies, which was a positive unexpected side-effect of the process.

Institutional use of the HIA
The local authority appears to have incorporated the HIA evidence into its policy formulation processes more than other stakeholders have done. A respondent from the local authority stated that the reason for this may be due to the local authority having greater ownership over the HIA: 'more ownership but the city council were different, they held (the) project management role ... for me there's something about a factor of success of the HIA is ownership of the project'. According to this individual, because the users of the HIA were also leading it, this was a factor in the successful institutionalisation of the HIA evidence.

HIA

In terms of the HIA findings and process being used, some responses to this question referred to the process of HIA itself, and how it results in workable outcomes. A respondent from the local authority stated that there were 'interesting outcomes but a pity that the power is so factionalised, and so it's hard to get action taken. Even in England, the councils have an input into planning, transport and roads and so it's easier to get action done and more productive, but in Northern Ireland it's different and power is fragmented'. According to this individual, the process of HIA was good and practicable, but the context within which the instrument is trying to infiltrate and influence, is fraught within political and administrative constraints. However, during the interviews conducted in phase II of this study, this issue of fragmented power is being resolved in the reform programme for local government, as for example, some planning and transport functions are being transferred to local authorities, including local development plan functions, which eases up the disjointed sectoral working relations of previous times.

A respondent of the Institute of Public Health stated that the HIA process on the Draft Air Quality Action Plan was a 'good example of getting statutory players around the table to work on the HIA, there was a positive shift in the attitude towards the HIA and the benefits that can come from it'. This was identified as a tangible outcome of the process, and one way in which the process itself was used.

Community

This respondent from the IPH also stated that this HIA case 'showed the use of engaging the community, who wouldn't be engaged in a normal process, and there were realistic recommendations which helped'. The fact that the community were engaged in the process, and are foreseen to use the evidence that comes from the HIA in future development and planning proposals, is deemed as a way that the HIA has been effectively used and has proven a useful instrument.

Part III: update on the Air Quality Action Plan HIA

There was no formal standalone evaluation conducted of the HIA on the Air Quality Action Plan, although according to statutory requirements the plan itself was monitored. Lavin and Metcalfe did review it as part of the European-wide assessment of HIA effectiveness in supporting decision-making (Wismar *et al.*, 2007). Lavin and Metcalfe (2007b) found that in relation to perceptions around effectiveness of the HIA for policy decision-making, those members who were involved in both the HIA and in developing the Air Quality Action

Plan were more positive and optimistic about the HIA being used in the plan, as opposed to mixed responses from those who took part in the HIA only.

Phase II interviews conducted in 2014 confirmed that the action plan which the HIA was conducted on finished substantially in 2010, and currently BCC is in the process of developing the next Air Quality Action Plan in collaboration with competent authorities and other partner organisations as is statutorily required. Respondents from the local authority reflected that more than likely there would not be an HIA explicitly conducted on this plan, although the council 'will be looking at health benefits of implementing any of the actions though we would not go as far as having an accompanying HIA to go along with it'. Reasons identified for not conducting an HIA this time around include the financial and resource restrictions in place as a result of the economic recession across the public administration and the 'lighter touch approach to policy' being promoted by the government. This emerging approach means that endeavours such as HIA would be supported more if they could be integrated into the regular (statutorily required) processes of consultation, instead of requiring a separate comprehensive HIA. This 'lighter touch approach' promoted by the government does not only apply or affect HIA, and as one respondent stated:

> (It's) not to say they're (government) setting aside health, the point is it mightn't stand as an HIA (that would be done as part of the upcoming action plan). Maybe the principles (of HIA) will be integrated into the normal consultation process, unlike last time we mightn't do something as elaborate as an HIA … (It will) simply be part of the consultation process, simply ask questions around the determinants of health.

In relation to the work of local authorities working in partnership with other agencies at local government and at central government levels, as a result of the local government reform there will be a transfer of planning and regeneration functions to the local authorities after the restructuring from April 2015 onwards. This will improve the abilities of local authorities to act and be involved in matters that affect air quality and other issues around environmental and health protection, however even after reform the DRD will still have responsibility for road transport matters. When asked if the reform of local government would have an impact on public health (and also this was asked of another respondent in phase II of the study as part of the second Northern Ireland HIA case (in Derry/Londonderry)), the following was one response:

> I think it's too early to say how these (reform) provisions will impact on public health and amalgamating councils is not due to take place until April next year (in 2015) and there's an plethora of activities going on to get these things in place. But overall the government statement is that a striving dynamic local government will create vibrant healthy communities. So health must be there at the centre with key local priorities, but it's too early to come back with an absolute

> statement, if you came back in two years time we'd be in a better position to respond on that.

Respondents felt that overall the reform agenda and provisions would result in more joined-up working across the sectors of transport, planning, housing, environment, health and so on. The community planning aspect of local government reform was highlighted as one measure that could allow HIA to advance once the reforms were instated after local authorities had amalgamated. This was also highlighted by a respondent from the Chartered Institute of Environmental Health Northern Ireland. Additionally, locally elected members of the council were identified as being much more aware of the determinants of health and the 'HiAP approach when taking decisions', as raised by a local authority respondent:

> It is positive, the council being more involved in community planning, the elected representatives are more *au fait* with how housing and road policies impact on health that they're taking decisions on. And I do think health is more widely considered across the council than it would have been previously.

In relation to HIA as an approach and instrument, a respondent from BHC in phase II of the study stated that there was a move away from conducting comprehensive HIAs and a move towards adopting a more pragmatic and flexible approach to integrating health considerations into policy-making. One of these ways was the move in Northern Ireland to promote a HiAP approach, which BHC and central government departments were working to integrate more into policy-making processes. BHC has developed a HiAP model which can be used in part or in whole, and HIA (in whole or elements of it) as an instrument which can advance the HiAP agenda. Once again, like with the development of the SIA in the RoI, one has to consider whether it matters or not the label we attribute to a particular tool or instrument, when the outcome (a consideration of health impacts of projects, programmes and policies) is what is realised ultimately. This pragmatic way of adopting a HIA approach to a local authority plan (Air Quality Action Plan) was identified as the probable way forward for now for local authorities, as identified by respondents from the local authority. The change in how HIA has developed in Northern Ireland was explored by a respondent from BHC, also in 2014:

> HIA is still on the agenda, but the visibility and delivery of it has changed slightly, I think we've moved away from the traditional comprehensive HIA to now using it as part of HiAP or health equity in all policies. Some people see that as one and the same thing, but we don't conduct HIAs the way in which we did 6 or 7 years ago. In NI there have been none completed recently. We've used the HIA approach in the HiAP work that we're doing with a number of government departments. They are not HIAs in the purest sense but integrate aspects of HIA.

HIA as an approach to tackle any lack of coordination across policy sectors and across governance tiers (between local and central) is not as strong as the Northern Ireland statutory duty on sustainable development, responsibility for which lies with the OFMDFM and which is better placed perhaps to promote an examination of how the determinants of health are affected by policies and how policies need to consider the determinants of health. According to the Northern Ireland (Miscellaneous Provisions) Act 2006 – article 25, which requires a public authority to, in exercising its functions, act in the way it considers best calculated to contribute to the achievement of sustainable development in Northern Ireland, except to the extent that it considers that any such action is not reasonably practicable in all the circumstances of the case coupled with compliance monitoring and reporting, is one mechanism to ensure greater whole-of-government working. It could also ensure that health is on the agenda when policies are being made and considered, than completing individual HIAs.

Lessons learned: public health, community participation and intersectoral working

The HIAs discussed in this chapter illustrate the way HIA can enable greater intersectoral partnership building and work with the goal to inform non-health sector policies of health impacts. Challenges associated with the cases discussed relate to the difficulties of working intersectorally, working with limited powers and functions at local government level, the impact of reform programmes and system restructuring, and tensions that continue to exist when organisations come together with their institutional priorities and assumptions underlying negotiations and work. The future for HIA as an approach and instrument may lie in it becoming more integrated into the planning processes in both jurisdictions, with the transfer of functions around planning and regeneration in local authorities and the development of the community planning initiative being the most promising examples of how this can happen. Also, it becoming integrated with HiAP approaches (as in NI) or part of the SIA in RoI, as an evolved approach and instrument, whereby elements are used in an organic way in order to be flexible and pragmatic for those seeking to adopt the approach towards building healthy public policies. This may work best as an approach to continuing HIA for as long as it exists without a legislative basis. As one respondent of BHC stated in an interview in 2014, 'I think the key elements of it has survived and it is (conducted) more as a part of the HiAP approach now. It is a more organic way of using it or doing it'. Perhaps the future for HIA will be for it to be adopted and integrated in parts as opposed to being conducted in its entirety which may cause a resource and financial burden on organisations that are not capable of supporting the process.

Community engagement was a strong element in both HIAs, through the direct engagement with individuals who would be affected by the Air Quality Action Plan (for instance, residents and primary schools) and transport and traffic initiatives (local residents), and continues to be a major feature in informing the policy process and those who are making the decisions, and informing those making key strategic decisions (in local authorities, for instance), as was illustrated by the Ballyfermot experience, in order to consider all possible effects and consequences. This point was succinctly summed up by one respondent from BCC in phase II of the study:

> It (HIA) was useful in defining health issues and concerns that maybe wouldn't be apparent to officers. Members of the public and other groups might know about them and they mightn't be noticeable to us, and it is useful in (showing) how people from different points of view approach different issues.

Conclusion

The HIA cases examined in this chapter illustrate the way that institutions (overarching structures) and values (underlying norms and beliefs) can impact on the way that HIA is viewed, conducted and ultimately used once it is completed. The HIAs were used to inform local policies and initiatives, and the degree to which they were used will be explored further in the final chapter, with a focus on the application of the conceptual lens and the generalisability of the findings.

Mittelmark *et al.* (2007) concluded that 'a community development approach to HIA can increase the likelihood that policy and decision-makers will listen when citizens raise issues of concern within their community' (Pursell and Kearns, 2012: 524). Tangible involvement of communities and a facilitation of their voices within the HIA process will enable some degree of empowerment and a way for communities to inform local policies, plans and initiatives that affect their daily lives. HIA will work in a maximised way if there is already strong community engagement and activity in an area before its commencement, as was the case in Dublin but not so much in the Belfast HIA. The HIAs were used in ways not foreseen, such as to inform and shape health promotion interventions in Ballyfermot in Dublin, and in facilitating greater awareness of the determinants of health across an array of partners in the Belfast HIA, much of which has remained with statutory officials working in the non-health sector in Belfast and as a vital evidence base connecting health and wellbeing with sectoral policies in transport, regional development, air quality and pollution and planning. Also, as was the case in Belfast, communities and partners involved in the process are in possession of evidence that they can use further down the line, to inform and shape initiatives and proposals, or in lobbying policy-makers on a variety of issues.

The lack of statutory recognition of HIA was also highlighted in the empirical research in this chapter as implying a value judgement from an institutional and central government policy level. If HIA is not established on a legislative basis, this inaction in itself reduces the credibility organisations and institutions may have in the approach and instrument. Also highlighted in this chapter was the motivation to initiate the HIAs. For many individuals and organisations, the HIA was seen as an instrument to ease out any strained intersectoral tensions or to 'convince' certain stakeholders from non-health backgrounds to adopt a more holistic approach to developing policies, taking account of the wider determinants of health. The extent to which HIA can be used as an implicit political means to a political end is an issue that was pertinently raised by some respondents in the cases and is an issue to be cognisant of when examining the underlying values, beliefs and motivations in conducting and using HIAs.

The following chapter continues with the story of HIA in RoI and NI based on empirical work, focusing primarily on one determinant of health (housing) among others that are evident within the process.

5

HIA in housing

Contentious and consensual

In a similar format as the previous chapter, this chapter starts off with an overview of the population health impacts of housing. Two HIAs are then described and explored using the conceptual lens as outlined in Chapter 2, as was done in Chapter 4. This chapter describes HIAs conducted in the topic of housing; one on the TAP, which is a local authority five-year plan for Traveller (Irish ethnic nomadic community) housing accommodation needs. The other HIA was performed on an urban regeneration project, specifically on the redesign of a social housing estate in Derry/Londonderry. The initiatives and plans that the HIAs were conducted on arose from Donegal County Council (local authority) and a housing proposal of the NIHE (strategic housing authority for the jurisdiction). A background description is given of each HIA (how and why they came about) and the story behind each HIA is explored. As a result of interviews conducted with participants on the HIA steering committees/groups representing all key stakeholders in the years 2007 and 2008 (local statutory bodies, local authority, community, public health, HIA experts and other local agencies) (phase I of the study), each case includes an exploration of the perspectives of the individuals sitting on each HIA's steering committees. An update of the impact of the HIAs is provided also as a result of a follow-up examination carried out in 2013 and 2014 (phase II of the study).

Housing and health impacts

A number of studies have examined the impact of housing on health and wellbeing. Lavin *et al.* (2006) emphasise the design issues of housing both in terms of the individual building and of the immediate environment, concluding that these physical and socio-economic factors impact on health. Housing has been found to be a greater determinant on health than any other factor, including lifestyle behaviours (Thomson *et al.*, 2003). Systematic reviews have been conducted examining the economic cost of health impacts of housing improvement schemes (Fenwick *et al.*, 2013) and of housing improvements on health (Morley, 2010). Blakely *et al.* (2011) conclude in their commentary ('Does housing policy impact health?') that although there is evidence to suggest the causation between health and housing, which aspect of housing and housing interventions improves health and wellbeing remains unclear. Another study, a systematic review examining housing improvements for health and socio-economic outcomes, found that housing investment which improves thermal comfort in the home can result in health improvements, and there is some evidence to suggest that better insulated homes can lead to fewer absences from work and school (Thomson *et al.*, 2013). HIAs of Roma housing policies in Europe found that housing had beneficial health effects when indoor and outdoor conditions, access to services and socio-economic conditions were improved. The HIAs found negative impacts could be estimated in relation to housing tenure and maintenance expenses (Molnar *et al.*, 2012). This brief overview of some of the scientific evidence available illustrates the causal linkages between housing design and conditions and overall health and wellbeing, which will be further illustrated in the following HIAs conducted on Traveller accommodation in RoI and on a social regeneration housing (improvement) project in NI.

HIA on a TAP, 2006 (Donegal, Republic of Ireland)

Part I: description

The Donegal Travellers Project (DTP) commissioned a retrospective comprehensive HIA on the TAP (2005 to 2008). The DTP is a community development project that represents the interests of Irish Travellers in County Donegal. The project was funded by the health services, the HSE. Given the poor quality of Traveller accommodation generally in the jurisdiction (Department of Social and Family Affairs, 2006; Department of Health, 2010), in County Donegal in this instance, conducting a HIA on local authority accommodation was viewed as an opportunity to introduce a stronger health dimension into the county's policy (Doyle, 2006). This is the first comprehensive HIA conducted in the Republic of Ireland on Traveller accommodation. The second Donegal County Council TAP (2005 to 2008), which was completed in 2004 and adopted in 2005, was an opportunity for the HIA to be carried out. The HIA aimed to assess the potential health impacts of the implementation of the TAP on the health of the population and to provide evidence-based recommendations so that the implementation would improve Traveller health in County Donegal. It was envisaged that the findings from the impact assessment process would be incorporated into the council's programme and policy plans, both concurrently and prospectively (Donegal Travellers Project, 2006). The impetus for conducting this HIA came from the DTP, which then garnered support from the HSE and finally with Donegal County Council. It was hoped that the HIA would reiterate and advocate to the council the links between health and housing, and the need for improved Traveller accommodation policy.

The Housing (Traveller Accommodation) Act was ratified in July 1998, requiring that local authorities, in consultation with the Travellers and Traveller representative organisations, formulate and adopt a five-year accommodation programme. Such TAPs are intended to ensure appropriate provision of accommodation to the Traveller communities and to guarantee the implementation of the measures of the programme (Silke, 2005). In general the TAPs are to be five years in duration although it can happen that they will be for four years. All local authorities had enacted such programmes from March 2000. As part of the 1998 legislation each council set up a Local Traveller Accommodation Consultative Committee (LTACC) so as to facilitate consultation between the housing authorities and Traveller communities.

An analysis was carried out in 2005 of the workability and the genuine consultation that arises from the LTACC. Both councillors and Traveller representatives, who participated in that study, did not believe productive and adequate consultation came from the LTACC. Councillors identified the culture of the institution (local authority) as having a pervading influence in the way council officials operated and dealt with Travellers and Traveller policy issues. The plans and TAPs are 'usually driven by professionals within the council who did not have a holistic view of the situation that councillors and community representatives have' (O Riain, 2005: 12). The negative attitude towards nomadism is felt to influence the operations and policies at local authority level. A recommendation from the 2005 report stated the necessity for 'a greater inter-agency dimension, bringing people with decision-making powers, together to address the issues' (O Riain, 2005: 13). Other recommendations included the need for independent chairs on committees dealing with Traveller accommodation. These suggestions were taken on board in this HIA case; an independent chair was appointed and the DTP advocated the Traveller way of life as unique to the county council officials during the process.

Poor health status is synonymous with this population group. Members of the Traveller community generally live shorter lives, living an average of eleven years less than the general population (Department of Health, 2010). The community experiences a higher infant mortality rate, higher early-school-leaver's rate and lower literacy levels when compared with the average of the Irish population (Department of Health, 2010). Health inequalities are starkly evidenced with this population group.

In this case, as opposed to the situation with the other three HIAs, the statutory bodies (specifically the local authority) were not the main instigators of the HIA but were intended as the main users of the HIA in policy. This then had important implications in terms of the user/owner dynamic in the use of HIA knowledge for policy development.

The HIA on Traveller Accommodation in Donegal was to facilitate the adoption of health knowledge into local council policy. A retrospective HIA was carried out, the timing of which would not allow findings and recommendations to be incorporated into the then ongoing five-year plan. However, it was expected that the HIA would be included in the development of specific detailed protocols in order to deliver the scheme on the ground, and according to interviews with county officials in 2014, the HIA was used in subsequent programmes.

The objectives of the HIA are as follows:

- To assess the potential health impacts of the implementation of the TAP on the health of the Traveller population.
- To produce evidence-based recommendations to implement the TAP in a way that would improve the health of the Traveller population in Donegal. (Doyle, 2006)

In addition, two unspecified yet expected outcomes from this HIA included the facilitation of the cross-sectoral collaboration on the issue of Traveller health and accommodation. The process was expected to inform all stakeholders of the health impacts of accommodation on the community.

Stakeholder involvement

For this HIA the main stakeholders included the HSE Western Area (health services), county council officials and Traveller organisations. An advisory group was established in early 2005 to oversee the conduct of the HIA. Representatives on this group were drawn from Donegal County Council, the HSE, DTP, the County Development Board, and the community and voluntary sector. One public health researcher was hired by the council in December 2004 to carry out the research.

In this Donegal HIA case study, eleven people were interviewed in phase I of the study (2007 and 2008) and four in 2014 (phase II). In phase I, a purposive sample of those on the advisory group was selected with follow-up interviews in phase II.

Donegal Travellers Project (DTP)

The DTP was initially established as a women's development project for a group of Traveller women in 1996, and then changed its focus to issues relating to the entire Travelling community in the environs of County Donegal in 1997. The DTP runs a number of different projects and programmes within its remit which aim to tackle social exclusion within the community. This project operates in partnership with the HSE in coordinating action on the ground with Traveller families and in tackling health inequalities through service provision.

Donegal County Council (DCC)
DCC is the local government authority for County Donegal. The housing services section of the council deals with requirements of the local populace in dealing with accommodation requests. The Director of Service, who is also the Assistant County Manager, represented the local authority on the HIA. This individual was therefore at a high level of power and influence in policy-making terms. In addition to this individual there was a social worker for Travellers on the advisory group.

Health Services Executive (HSE)
The HSE supports the DTP through the North West Traveller Health Unit and in particular the work of the Primary Health Care Project. The Social Inclusion team of the HSE Western Area is the relevant unit that operates in partnership with the DTP. The work ethos of the HSE staff would draw from the rationale of working from the All-Ireland Traveller Health Study (2010). On the HIA advisory group there were three individuals representing the views of the HSE organisation.

Donegal County Development Board and the Donegal Local Development Company (DLDC)
Both of these organisations play a key part in the enterprise and community life of County Donegal. The Donegal Local Development Company, known in the locality as the DLDC, delivers twelve EU and Irish government funded programmes that are centred on local development and community enterprise matters (DLDC, 2007). One representative from each of these organisations had a place on the advisory group, although respondents described their role as 'peripheral' compared to the local authority, health services and DTP stakeholders.

Expert HIA practitioner/researcher
An independent HIA researcher was hired to lead on the methodological procedures of this process, and to compile the relevant data for the HIA, drawing from both qualitative and quantitative sources.

Community Workers Cooperative
Donegal Community Workers Cooperative (CWC) was formed in 1994. The aim of the network is to implement social change by conducting policy analysis of local and national strategies, in order to ascertain where and how social

action can be taken for the wellbeing of the socio-economic good of the locality (Community Workers Cooperative, 2007). An independent chairperson was brought into the process at later stages in the HIA from the CWC, in order to facilitate the process and deal with the disagreement that had developed between the DTP and county council officials.

HIA methodology

The Merseyside Guidelines were followed for the completion of this HIA (Scott-Samuel *et al.*, 1998), with a mixture of qualitative and quantitative methods employed. This was a collaborative project, whereby the HIA researcher worked closely with the DTP community health workers. This group guaranteed a 'gateway' into the population group. A quantitative survey was formulated with the literacy and educational needs of Travellers kept in mind. The community health workers (members of the Traveller community) received training and proceeded to conduct the fieldwork in the summer of 2005. There was a 64 per cent response rate. This data was correlated with the interviews held with residents of halting sites and with evidence from the literature review, to result in the main findings of the HIA.

HIA outcomes

A number of findings arose from this HIA on Traveller accommodation. Some of the most important findings are indicated below:

- Most people view improved accommodation conditions as key to improved health.
- Poor living conditions are the main reasons for differences in health between groups of Travellers.
- Health problems are more common among children living in homes with problems with cold and damp.
- Poor living conditions are concentrated in current temporary site accommodations.
- Stress levels are high amongst all groups in this research; stress is mainly due to living conditions with site residents.

The health impacts of accommodation policy, as researched in this study, can be categorised in two ways; physical health (as indicated above) and mental health (stress levels and the anxiety associated with societal exclusion).

A Health Impact Analysis was carried out in order to map the commitments made in the TAP against the positive and negative health impacts of this HIA. Although the statements of action in the programme are positive overall, there is much political rhetoric on the issue. Recommendations for the HIA were developed over the duration of three workshops, carried out in late 2005/

early 2006. Although recommendations were agreed upon, the implementation and adoption of them in decision-making circles remained the challenge. Given the politically and socially controversial nature of the topic (Travellers and accommodation), the assimilation of evidence into decision-making within the council and HSE was testing. The continuation of multi-sectoral working and partnership on this issue of Traveller health and accommodation is key for the findings of the HIA to be incorporated and 'heard' within the policy formulation processes. This has been reaffirmed in the phase II part of the study (interviews carried out in 2014).

Policy process for the Traveller Accommodation HIA

The fundamental goal of this HIA was to evaluate the potential impacts on health of the TAP, and to formulate recommendations for the implementation of the programme by using the findings from the IA process. It was envisaged that findings would be used as part of the national Traveller Health study to be carried out in the near future, and by the HSE and Donegal County Council when formulating policies and services for the Traveller community.

Part II: analysis

Interviews conducted with respondents for this Donegal HIA case were analysed and the results of this analysis are presented in the next section. The conceptual lens, as outlined in Chapter 2, provides a framework for presenting the findings from the interview data. In this Donegal case study, eleven people were interviewed for phase I (2007 and 2008), and four for phase II (2014).

'Institutions matter': New Institutional Theory

Are institutions ready? The timing of HIA as a policy support tool

The timing of HIA as a policy support tool was asked during the interviews in order to explore the perspective of those on the HIA advisory group, which included both decision-makers of statutory bodies and members of the community.

One respondent from the local authority stated that yes, the time is right to use knowledge and evidence that comes from HIAs. Four respondents from the HSE, CWC and HIA researcher stated that 'maybe' the time was right to use HIAs. These individuals were uncertain as to the timing of HIAs based on their experience; unsure as to whether their time had come to be used for policy. One HSE respondent stated that the time may not be right for all, alluding to the fact that certain stakeholders, and the institutions they come from, may not be ready. This individual had no qualms in saying that, in the opinion of this respondent, Donegal County Council was not ready to use HIAs at the present time. The respondent from the CWC stated that perhaps the time was right, but it depended on the political will of the council.

Normative dimension: do institutions shape behaviour?

The use of Institutional Theory in this study was to establish the extent of the influence certain institutions have on the use of HIAs and the knowledge that came from them which was intended to inform policy. Those interviewed in this case were stakeholders in the HIA process, and were on the advisory group as representatives of their relevant bodies, be it from a local authority (Donegal County Council), health service (HSE) or the community perspective (DTP, community representative). The responses to this section were grouped in thematic categories. First, at institutional, HIA process and policy process levels, a number of constraining factors upon behaviour were found. Second, the nature of Traveller policy and the impact this has upon the use of HIAs in policy was elicited from the data. Third, ideas and values played a constraining role in this case study, in the use of HIAs.

An issue came up in this case study that has arisen in other instances, as is evidenced in the HIA literature. An issue of the owner/user dynamic was clearly evident in this HIA on Traveller accommodation. The main driver (owner) of the HIA was not also the main user of the HIA in policy. This is to say, the DTP were the convenors and instigators of the HIA, and they organised the conduct of the research. However, it was Donegal County Council that was envisioned to use the HIA knowledge and evidence once the process had been completed. Therefore, in this instance, there was no symbiotic relationship between owner and user of the HIA, and this may have been a factor in its implementation of process and recommendations.

One respondent from the HSE alluded to this point, as indicated in the following:

> It is more difficult when it wasn't in one organisation; it was a voluntary organisation and two statutory organisations. And also maybe that it was one organisation carrying out the research but the recommendations related more to another organisation, that was a difficult situation as well.

The institution (Donegal County Council) that was envisioned to use the HIA was perceived by the DTP as 'a big barrier anyway before it started. They considered this an attack on their policy, for them to implement (the HIA's recommendations) they'd have to have big changes in their policy'. The feeling around the local authority was undeniably negative, as evidenced from all interviewees (except the council officials) during data collection. Institutional constraints from the perspective of this interviewee from the DTP depended on which agency the HIA would impact most on; this was a confounding factor in the successful process and use of the HIA in policy.

One respondent from the local authority stated that this HIA was the first one completed on Traveller accommodation in Ireland and no other local authority had yet been involved in one. This individual was proud that it had been carried out, as the HIA being conducted at all was an achievement in his opinion despite the ongoing usefulness of the document and process. This issue has also been highlighted in the following section where an update on the HIA is given.

The respondent from the CWC highlighted the fact that there were staffing issues constraining the process of the HIA, and the way that people worked and behaved. It was clear that those interviewed for this case study were more than aware of the institutional constraints upon individual behaviour and action. In addition to this overarching influence upon behaviour regarding the HIA and the subsequent use of it, there were also influences at HIA and policy process levels.

At the level of the conducting of the HIA process, amalgamation of evidence and recommendations, and subsequent assumed use for informed policy, there were misunderstandings at play. Most notably, among certain stakeholders on the advisory group, there was a lack of understanding of what the HIA would be about as HIA was a novel instrument introduced at the time. It therefore required a great deal of explanation to all those envisioned to be part of the process, before it commenced.

From the perspective of the policy process and the use of the HIA in it, a number of factors impacting upon this use were highlighted in the interviews. The respondent from the local authority was quite confident that the HIA would be used: 'we'll be informed by the HIA, we will be, we have to be, we're part of that so we will be.' This use of the HIA was discussed in the context of the next Traveller Accommodation Plan; plans for which commenced in 2009.

The HIA researcher stated that there are definitely institutional constraints upon the use of HIAs 'because there's so many (constraints) on Traveller policy and the room for manoeuvre for decision makers is limited because of the hostility towards Travellers'. The limitations upon decision-makers in the formulation of policy were highlighted by this researcher and the hostility alluded to here is present across the entire society.

The respondent from the CWC pointed out that the local authority, which was envisioned as the main user of the HIA, both in the ongoing formulation of Traveller accommodation policy, and in the delivery of services to the group, 'haven't enough (people) working from a community perspective, which is a problem'. The different approach of working which the HIA entailed (collaboration with the community; a bottom-up community development approach) is not one used regularly at local authority level in its daily workings, and so would have proven difficult for its employees on the HIA to adapt to the different mode of practice.

Finally a point was raised by a respondent from the HSE regarding the need for political and managerial commitment to the HIA process: 'if you don't have buy-in to the idea of the HIA, there is a risk that it is just a paper exercise or a research exercise, and that the follow through that you expect won't materialise.' This point highlights the need for the espousal of all stakeholders in the process, and support from their relevant institutions is also necessary.

In particular, Traveller accommodation policy …

It was evident during the gathering of data for this case that the area of Traveller policy, especially regarding accommodation policy, was highly contentious. This controversial nature of the policy topic, where animosity and resentment breed fiercely across society, acted as a barrier to the use of the HIA conducted on the TAP.

Political dimension: do politics matter?

This study looked at the influence of such a political dimension, by asking the respondents about their opinions on the extent that politics were at play between the varying interests during the process of the HIA.

The responses to this question include reflections on the political dimension at a micro-level (individuals) and macro-level (institutions), the perception of politics, politics and polarised attitudes and positions regarding the area of Traveller work, and the issue of HIA requiring statutory recognition.

Individuals: the gatekeepers to the institutions (withholding the keys?)

In response to the question of politics, many interviewees focused attention upon the different interests involved in the HIA, on the advisory group. It was clear that at an individual level, many interviewees felt that other stakeholders brought with them an element of tension and misunderstanding, as evidenced by their behaviour and actions.

A respondent from the HSE involved in the process stated that the workings of the HIA were too complicated: 'if an ordinary person like me doesn't understand what's going on, there's something wrong.' This statement was further qualified by the same individual, by stating that there were definite problems on the advisory group, because of what people were saying, not saying, and saying with double meanings and intentions; points of view were not being stated upfront. This will be further illustrated in a following paragraph.

With regard to the advisory group, a number of interviewees pointed out some prohibitive behaviours that were noted by some members of the HIA; there were 'delaying tactics at the meetings' (DTP respondent); 'people not showing up for meetings' (DTP respondent); 'just things that weren't being said (upfront), you know, if people could have said "no" or "there's difficulty in progressing with that" but when people don't say things like that there's a difficulty' (HSE respondent); 'a lot of politics, a lot of back benching' (DTP health worker respondent).

Due to the varying degrees of commitment and agreement on the advisory group, an independent chairperson was introduced to the HIA halfway through the process. The reasoning behind this action was to introduce an impartial person, who was deemed acceptable by both polarised sides on the HIA (the Traveller organisation on the one hand, the statutory bodies on the other, in particular the county council), into the process. At the time that this individual was introduced, a stalemate had been reached on the advisory group; such was the disagreement and discord between the different stakeholders.

A respondent from the local authority, when asked about the politics on the HIA advisory group, noted that a wide variety of people came to the table with different outlooks. He did not specify that there were any politics at play, but simply noted that there was a certain amount of tension given the array of perspectives in the HIA process. This individual explained that it was inevitable that people would come to the process with different perspectives. However, there was little indication in this interview of the tension, strife, disquiet and disagreement amongst all stakeholders, in particular in disagreement with authority officials, which other respondents discussed in response to this question. This reflection illustrates how the same story can be viewed with different eyes and from different viewpoints.

Institutions: the gate and the building

In discussing the degree and nature of politics and conflicting interests in this HIA, some interviewees focused on the statutory bodies (local authority and health services). A respondent from the DTP stated that senior people from the local authority primarily, and from the health services, were needed so that any recommendations agreed during the HIA could be taken back to the relevant institution to be adopted and used in their respective institutions.

It was felt by the researcher that the council was 'paying lip service' and that it had 'no intention that any real decisions would come out'. This negativity towards the council was reverberated, although in varying degrees, throughout all interviews, except those involving council officials. However, this resistance in cooperation may have been related to the institutional constraints facing the individuals rather than any personal animosity in the HIA. The chairperson stated that, while acknowledging and recognising the sometimes defensiveness of the council officials, such officials are accountable to the elected representatives of Donegal County Council, and their actions and statements in the HIA were reflective of this relationship. The chairperson pointed out that 'all politics is local in Donegal' and 'there's a lot of resistance around Traveller accommodation, and restrictions on budgets at the moment would impact on the area of Traveller work', which impacted on the HIA process.

Stakeholders in the process were overall deemed as helpful from the HSE institution by the respondent from the CWC. However, this individual qualified this statement by reflecting that 'a lot of good people came to it (the HIA), they were well meaning, especially the HSE who were driving the agenda. Individuals in the HSE, maybe, it mightn't reflect the ethos of the organisation, it might just be that the individuals we dealt with were particularly good'.

A respondent from the HSE stated that staffing issues and procedures at an institutional level within the local authority became an issue: 'problems arose, like the turnover of staff and gaps in the staffing was an issue for this HIA'.

The perception of politics

It is beyond any doubt that in this HIA, politics and tensions were endemic from beginning to end, and played a role in the process, the formulation of recommendations, and the subsequent use of the HIA in policy.

Interviewees reiterated this in their reflective discussions. A HSE respondent stated that there were 'a lot of politics ... with a small p and big P ... I couldn't see the path forwards in the HIA in the advisory group because of the politics there'. Due to the tension between the stakeholders, and the history of conflict between the voluntary and statutory interests on the topic in the area, the HIA was actually used as a tool to break down such negative history and resentments; the HIA was used to cut through the politics. This point was highlighted by the HIA researcher:

> Used the HIA to cut through the politics, it was the hope that if they discussed health it would break down barriers and depoliticise the issues on Traveller accommodation needs.

Controversies, adversaries and resentments: working on Traveller accommodation

As indicated in the previous section, there was a legacy of conflict in the area of work in Traveller accommodation in County Donegal, between the DTP and the local authority in particular. This 'history of confrontation ... was in the room and in the process' and the 'baggage from previous encounters' acted as a barrier to the workings of the HIA. Although it was hoped the HIA would prevent this 'baggage' from becoming a problem, this aspect interfered to a large extent with the way that the HIA was perceived by the council, and the way that it was presented by the DTP. The former body viewed the HIA with scepticism, viewing it as a mechanism that the Traveller representative body would use to attack the policy of the council. The latter body went into the process with the intention of presenting the facts and evidence of the HIA, which would prove that the accommodation policy of the local authority was providing sub-standard services that led to poor health of Travellers. Undeniably, the two groups, at polar opposite sides of the policy spectrum, were bound to clash. The fact that it was within the space of the HIA was irrelevant, as the subject area of Traveller accommodation was controversial.

On the advisory group there was a certain amount of 'controversy over the wording of terms', in particular the use of 'anti-racism' (DTP respondent). The context of this issue was in relation to anti-racism training that the DTP provides on an ongoing basis to statutory bodies. The DTP questioned whether it may be provided during this HIA process. During this interview, it was pointed out that for a number of years such training has been provided to the HSE, without any defensive reaction or controversy. However, when the suggestion for such training was brought up with the local authority officials, they rejected it as they felt they were being called racist and anti-Traveller. This example illustrates the fraught tension that was embedded in the process, and the quick-fire reactions with regard to issue around Traveller practice and policy.

The respondent from the local authority, when asked about the political dimension in this HIA, acknowledged that some people came to the process 'with prejudice and fear, some with attitudes that don't value the ethnic value of Travellers. There are always those things at play when there's a cross-section of people'. This individual did not specify who was coming to the proverbial table with such attitudes and fears.

HIA: must become mandatory, not remain voluntary

A respondent from the HSE, in response to the question on the political dimension, stated that until HIAs are statutory, there will always be a problem with them and conflicting interests will continue to interfere in the process. This individual acknowledged that with statutory recognition for HIA, would come about a certain standardisation and it would not matter what the subject area of the HIA was, or who the stakeholders were in the impact assessment.

The role of value judgements in the HIA process

The values dealing with Travellers as a minority group made up the bulk of responses to this question on value judgements. The impact of miscommunication of values and assumptions during the HIA was raised repeatedly during the interviews. The lack of understanding of the holistic concept of health that is at the core of the HIA technique also indicated some conflicting values held by stakeholders in the process, which in turn resulted in a conflict of the main values that HIAs hold true.

Values and Travellers

Values, attitudes and beliefs around the Traveller community arose during the data collection phase for this case study. The values placed upon the community by all stakeholders in the process, from the statutory and voluntary representative groups, played a key role in the HIA process and in the use of HIA knowledge thereafter.

The biggest stumbling block is the lack of recognition of the community in statute: 'there is no statutory acknowledgement of the travelling community as an ethnic community' in either local or national policy, and this is a cause for controversy at any meetings between the voluntary group (DTP) and state agencies (the county council, which is the local housing authority, and the HSE, providing health services) (DTP respondent). It was 'like an elephant in the room, whether Travellers are an ethnic minority or not'. There's immediately a 'clash of belief systems around Traveller definition', which affects any collaborative working between the agencies as both points of view are polarised and entrenched (DTP respondent). This issue was bound to affect the process and use of the HIA, and it did.

An interviewee explained that there was a lot of tension at meetings, and there were very revealing comments being made, for instance:

> Planners might say something, or even public health workers, would vocalise those attitudes, saying things like 'well what do you expect from them' or 'it's their own fault for doing that', 'they bring it on themselves', things like that.

It was clear that the prejudices and fears that mainstream society hold towards the Travelling community were mirrored in the interactions between the statutory bodies and the representative community agency. It was a reflection of the real story that exists for the community in society. In meetings, stakeholders were talking down to the Travellers, 'criticising them … the process did show up that values made a huge difference' (HSE respondent). Finding a 'common space was very very difficult' (HSE respondent) in meetings, yet there was a strained 'politics of politeness' as both the Traveller voluntary agency and the statutory bodies were keen to attempt to work the HIA process as best as possible (DTP respondent).

The DTP recognised that it was a 'politically based organisation, we have very clear values and beliefs in terms of what we want to achieve as an organisation, and for us we have our baggage too', as would the statutory authorities. However, entrenched views on the HIA advisory group led to an impenetrable impasse, as there are 'people who see housing as the best option (for Travellers) and that's it' (HSE respondent). An immovable stalemate of clashing attitudes and values illustrated clearly what a 'difficult area of work Traveller accommodation is, as every person comes from a different perspective and I suppose people don't know what it's like to be a Traveller' (local authority respondent).

Value judgements

Respondents were keenly aware of the role that values played in this HIA, most notably in relation to the subject of the HIA, as opposed to the IA technique and process itself, however. One respondent stated that there were 'a lot of underlying value judgements, although the value judgements were not around the HIA but attributable to Travellers and the impression was that the attitude of the settled community was very prevalent in the minds of the policy-makers'. Clearly the subject area of Traveller accommodation, and the context of the policy area, took precedence in the HIA, over the actual impact assessment process itself.

Social determinants of health

It was noted by the public health researcher that there was a 'reluctance to engage with the concept of social determinants of health' by some of the statutory stakeholders. This lack of common ground and common understanding of some of the fundamental issues and values at the core of HIA became problematic during the HIA meetings, as this difference of opinion and understanding arose. A more holistic conceptualisation of health, however, is not wholly accepted or known on the part of non-health sector individuals throughout RoI. Perhaps in time the wider determinants of health can become more established and accepted.

Miscommunication

A major issue that repeatedly came up throughout all the interviews, was the role that 'miscommunication' played in the HIA process, both on the advisory group and outside the meeting rooms. A respondent from the HSE noted that, stating that 'people coming from different perspectives were not the problem, but it's that it's not communicated … But if we don't communicate that then it's difficult to find a way forward, going around in circles'. It certainly seems that, from an objective viewpoint, better communication of values, opinions and positions, would have resulted in a more open, transparent and productive process for the HIA to operate.

It is also important to note that HIA is a novel approach and may not be fully understood, which may have added to the lack of communication/miscommunication issue, as a respondent from the local authority noted:

> I don't think it's been fully understood … We're in there, with the HSE and the people who run the working group are in the HSE as well so we carry it forward from that perspective. The DTG certainly would be driving it, driving us to meet the recommendations. On a wider field, it's something we have to develop yet.

Knowledge use for policy development

Regarding the use of the HIA in policy development, respondents were asked to reflect on the extent, as far as they knew, that the HIA was used in policy and how useful was the HIA to local policy development processes.

HIA recommendations

In response to this question on knowledge use, the overall consensus was that 'some of them (recommendations) were taken on board, some not'. The recommendations were deemed as being realistic 'but some people didn't think so', referring to the local county council in this instance, according to a HSE respondent. Agreeing on the recommendations took a greater length of time than the entire data collection period for the HIA. Such was the stalemate, lack of agreement and entrenchment of positions on the advisory group. There was much negativity and disappointment with this HIA, as 'we did a lot of work, and it was diluted by the council' in the formulation and adoption of recommendations according to a respondent from the HSE.

From the perspective of the local authority, the HIA was deemed as useful but would have to be considered within the 'bigger picture' of Traveller work and what the council can and cannot achieve. In the recommendations, it was noted by this individual that there were a number issues that were done, being done, or too early to be carried out. There were a number of spin-offs, intangible benefits, which arose from the HIA. For instance, the community health workers of the DTP were now skilled in interviewing skills and could participate in the upcoming national Traveller health study. Findings from the HIA on children's health were used as part of a workshop in September 2005, highlighting the impact of housing on health. The HIA was used in many respects, as a respondent from the HSE noted: 'we used the findings of the HIA, and that wouldn't have happened at all, or it wouldn't have happened as fast if the findings of the HIA weren't there, so there were spin-offs from it, exactly.'

Institutions

In response to the question on the HIA recommendations, some interviewees state that institutional rules, processes and standards acted as a barrier to the use of the HIA, and 'maybe would be better to use when statutory' (HSE respondent). In addition to this point, the need for political and managerial buy-in and commitment to the idea of HIA is a necessary ingredient if the HIA is to be used for the purpose it was elicited. Indeed, as one interviewee pointed out, recommendations would be used if there was strong organisational and institutional commitment to the HIA. If this is missing, then the recommendations and what they entail are meaningless (DTP respondent).

Policy process

In relation to the policy process, and the use of the HIA to inform policy, a number of issues arose regarding the utilisation of the recommendations.

A respondent from the HSE believed that there was a lack of understanding of the tool by policy-makers, even by the end of the process, which inhibited the use of the HIA: 'I don't think there's a full appreciation of it, even from policy-makers, I don't think there's an understanding what it's all about.'

The researcher noted that the HIA may not be 'immediately useful for policy, maybe it's a brick in the wall towards something more substantial, it started as a process and may show results down the road'. The HIA may have an indirect impact that may require further examination over a longer term period. This was partially the case in that the HIA was part of the TAP (2009–13) and referred to in the subsequent TAP (2014–18). The extent to which the recommendations have been implemented throughout these subsequent programmes is highly debated.

The researcher also pointed out that there was an 'overwhelming negativity attributed to the area by the decision makers, there was a real "not in my back yard" mentality coming from them. There's a vicious cycle of hostility and it came from the Travellers too'. The attitudes of those making policy affect the way in which such evidence is viewed and used in policy.

Collaboration and partnership

Due to the nature of HIAs, partnership and cross-sectoral working was integral to the success of the project. In relation to this case specifically, some interviewees focused on the issue of collaboration, partnership and inter-agency consultation, in both positive and negative light.

A respondent from the local authority stated that there was a lot of 'good collaboration and yet on the ground a lot of difficulties too'. With regard to difficulties this individual was referring to difficulties with working with the Travelling community on issues of security and in working with the Gardaí on such issues. Such difficulties were not directly related to the HIA but played a part in enhancing tension at the meetings, and went some way to explain such tensions. As has been stated already in this section, this Traveller accommodation HIA was set within a myriad of problems and issues of working on accommodation and with the community. However, good collaboration did come out of the HIA. Indeed, it is miraculous the extent of agreement around the final recommendations that came from the HIA, because of the degree of friction and discord during the process.

The LTACC has used the HIA in its work, and also refers to it as a method of good practice in fostering collaboration and intersectoral working on Traveller issues, according to the CWC respondent.

However, it is undeniable that 'participation with stakeholders was difficult' and the degree of hostility coming from the statutory and voluntary agencies on certain matters relating to Traveller policies and accommodation (researcher respondent). Although the HIA does require collaboration and partnership, in certain contexts it can be difficult. This HIA on Traveller accommodation policy is one such context.

Political will

Regarding the recommendations, some interviewees did point to the fact that political and managerial 'will isn't there to implement them, and the steering group isn't there to push it' (DTP respondent). The commitment to implement and use the HIA recommendations needs to be in place. Otherwise, the HIA will gather dust on the shelves of various institutions, never used. One interviewee pointed out that it 'all depends on an individual's will and their power to act'. The will and drive to act must come from key senior individuals in relevant tiers of power in relevant institutions. Without such key people, the utilisation of the HIA, and the implementation of the recommendations, is uncertain, as is clear from this case study. The chairperson of the HIA stated that the process and the outcome recommendations and findings were useful but without commitment, they could fall by the wayside, never to be used or referred to again.

HIA process

The process of the HIA was considered a 'very interesting process', as stated by a respondent from the HSE and as communicated by many others who were interviewed.

However there was 'a lot of negative feeling around the HIA', both during its conduct and in the aftermath. According to a HSE respondent, the process could be compared to a relationship break up. The respondent reflected on the feeling of wasted time, energy, resources, and of disappointment and frustration, as expressed by an individual deeply involved in the HIA from beginning to end. The respondent also reflected on the importance of key individuals in key positions of power who have an attitude of commitment and motivation for the HIA. Such individuals also are referred to as 'policy entrepreneurs' or 'HIA champions' in the HIA academic and research community (O'Mullane and Quinlivan, 2012). They are identified as necessary ingredients in the conduct of HIAs, and just as importantly, in the use of them once they are completed.

A respondent from the CWC described how the HIA report was launched by the Minister for Health and Children at the time. A big event was planned for the HIA; it was a highly politicised event in order to garner support and direct attention towards the HIA on the TAP. The extent to which this event garnered such support is questionable, as explored by this respondent, but it was a well organised event and did illustrate the importance the stakeholders in the process attributed to the process and outcome document.

Part III: update on the TAP HIA

An official evaluation of the TAP HIA (2006) has not been conducted. Since no formal evaluation was carried out on the HIA, and because of the divergence of opinions on the implementation of the HIA recommendations, respondents from the HSE and the local authority completed short evaluation surveys. The survey listed the twenty-three recommendations from the HIA and sought clarification of their implementation, which were rated as being implemented; not implemented; partially; not known. The recommendations included commitments from the TAP that would positively impact on the health of the Traveller group, and there was some consensus on these three commitments being in the TAP and implemented. However, for the remaining twenty recommendations, there was direct divergence and only an in-depth evaluation of the HIA would illustrate whether in fact the recommendations have been implemented, partially, or not at all. This is not the purpose of this book, to provide such an evaluation. It is very clear, however, that the TAP HIA is perceived in different ways by the stakeholders who were involved, and will hopefully stimulate continued future work on the health status of Travellers in the county. O'Mullane and Quinlivan (2012), in their examination of the role that local government plays within HIAs being conducted and being used for policy development, found that the TAP HIA could be classified as an oppositional case. It was initiated in order to bring greater awareness of health inequalities experienced by Traveller families in County Donegal to local authority officials and to ensure the TAP would be more health-promoting and health-protective for the community. It was the underlying motive of some stakeholders involved in this HIA to oppose the then accommodation policy direction which was not considered by various stakeholders to be Traveller-centred or culturally appropriate. It was a worthy endeavour to conduct this HIA. However, with an incredibly sensitive topic such as accommodation and the Traveller community, this HIA faced challenges before it had even begun. The success of the HIA in terms of its recommendations being implemented is considered by respondents as either poor or excellent (both views were expressed in interviews with respondents from the DTP, HSE and local authority in 2014 and within the surveys completed as mentioned previously). There appears to be a great disconnect within this HIA.

Was the HIA used to inform policy development? Yes, if you consider that it has been referred to and included in the TAP document as an appendix (2009–13) and yes, as it was named as a relevant policy document in this current (at the time of writing) TAP (2014–18). It is true that the discourse legacy of the HIA has continued within the pertinent policy documents. It was the first HIA conducted on the TAP in the jurisdiction and by the time of writing, the only one. This shows a commendable amount of cross-sectoral thinking and innovation on the part of the stakeholders involved in the HIA. This HIA provided, tactically and technically, a space for reasoning and discussion 'to navigate facts, values and processes underlying the substantive and procedural dimensions of policy' (Harris *et al.*, 2014: 1). However the expectations of the process on the part of the stakeholders involved varied and were often incompatible with one another.

Recommendations of the HIA are considered to have been included in the TAPs by the local authority, but not by the DTP and HSE which continue to be part of the consultative process in developing the five-year plans. The stakeholders involved in the HIA have opposing views as to what defines the success of this HIA. The assumptions underlying the HIA were that it sought to influence the development of more Traveller appropriate accommodation, 'to change the minds of the local authority', whereas the local authority is focused on implementing statutory obligations in as consultative a way as is possible, is focused on the fundamental task of housing people, without necessarily ensuring that the accommodation is always strictly culturally appropriate. The local authorities in the RoI take their direction and lead from the decisions made in the elected members' chamber and from the laws of the land agreed in the national parliament. In this respect, the TAPs are designed and delivered in order to provide housing and services. For this purpose, the TAPs have been fulfilling their goal. How they are regarded, delivered, received, in which way the Traveller community perceives the services and accommodation offers, and the perception of the cultural-appropriateness of the services being offered, is often what causes the tension between some statutory bodies, the community and representative community groups.

As concluded by O'Mullane (2009a) and O'Mullane and Quinlivan (2012), the HIA was conducted on a challenging and highly sensitive topic, in a society that generally views Traveller culture and behaviour in a negative light (Department of Health, 2010). This negativity towards the community cannot be overemphasised. Within this societal context, it is not surprising that the HIA has been viewed so disparately by the partners who worked together in the original HIA advisory group. In order to ensure that the HIA recommendations within the TAP have explicitly been implemented in practice, a full-scale evaluation could be conducted of the HIA and a monitoring group could be set up to evaluate the longer-term impact of the HIA.

HIA of NIHE proposal to redevelop Dove Gardens estate, 2005 (Derry/Londonderry, Northern Ireland)

Part I: description

A comprehensive prospective HIA on a NIHE proposal to redevelop an estate in the Brandywell electoral ward in Derry/Londonderry city was conducted in 2005 and 2006. This is the first prospective HIA on housing redevelopment in either jurisdiction. The findings of the HIA have influenced the structural shape of the redevelopment. The agency that led the implementation of the HIA was

Cooperation and Working Together (CAWT), a cross-border health and social care initiative. CAWT was established in 1992 when the health boards working along the geographical border between the RoI and NI signed the Ballyconnell Agreement. The Ballyconnell Agreement (Ireland) was signed in July 1992 between the North Eastern Health Board/North Western Health Board (RoI), and the Southern Health and Social Services Board and the Western Health and Social Services Board (NI). This agreement signified commitment on the part of these formerly called health boards (health services) to work together to improve the health and wellbeing of their populations (Glackin and Farrell, 2006). This housing HIA was part financed by the EU through INTERREG III 'A Programme for Ireland' (2000 to 2006), under measure 3.2 (health and wellbeing).

The story of this HIA started when CAWT was approached by the West Area Planner from the NIHE to consider conducting a HIA of a housing regeneration project planned for Derry/Londonderry city. This was agreed upon by CAWT and NIHE, and the government Departments of Health in both the Republic and Northern Ireland were approached for support and permission to proceed.

Dove Gardens is a council housing estate on the periphery of the Bogside and is less than one mile from Derry/Londonderry city centre. It is made up of seventy-six dwellings that were built in 1966. Deficiencies of the Dove Gardens estate were established by the NIHE Project Team in 2003, which was set up to develop proposals for redevelopment of the area.

The following are some of the problems with the housing, which arose from the team's investigation:

- Communal access: via open public stairwells and deck.
- No defensible space: there was little space between the residents' front door and the street. The front doors of the upper story maisonettes open directly onto the public deck.
- Poor clothes drying and waste disposal facilities: Bin chutes and clothes drying areas were communal, which created a health hazard. Drying areas were deemed insecure and unsafe at night. (Glackin and Farrell, 2006: 9)

Dove Gardens was originally built for small to medium sized families. However, household composition in 2004 showed that 80 per cent of households were made up of single occupants or small family units. The living space was unsuitable for the then current population demographic profile.

There are a number of reasons why the HIA in the Dove Gardens estate was carried out. Primarily, the residential community exists in one of the most deprived of Northern Ireland (Northern Ireland Statistics and Research Agency, 2005; Bonner, 2007) and was to benefit from the HIA process. The estate was known locally as 'Beirut', due to its run-down appearance and reputation for crime and anti-social behaviour (Bonner, 2007). Just 1 per cent of the population went on to third level education (Bonner, 2007), which illustrates the picture of social inequality experienced within the community (Bonner, 2011). The housing proposal would be influenced at its design stage, so that the findings of the HIA would be considered in the planning of the regeneration scheme. The HIA would add to the evidence-base correlating health and housing, and would inform decision-makers of this wider issue. In addition, the HIA was aimed to improve cross-sectoral cooperation and provide 'a structural framework for investigation and discussion of health impacts and the identification of more impacts compared to not doing one' (Glackin and Farrell, 2006: 10).

The purpose of this HIA was to increase the awareness of health implications of the regeneration programme in the Dove Gardens estate. The steering group of the HIA developed the objectives of the project, as follows:

- To influence the design for the regeneration of Dove Gardens.
- To improve the health and wellbeing of people living in Dove Gardens and surrounding areas.
- To promote community participation to enable local communities to contribute to, and influence, the decision-making processes as they impact on their community.
- To communicate the work of the steering group to all stakeholders in the regeneration project. (Glackin and Farrell, 2006: 12)

The objectives were decided upon at the scoping stage of the HIA, which is the second stage in the IA process.

Stakeholder involvement

There were a number of stakeholders in the process. CAWT, NIHE and members of the Health Action Zone 'Investing for Health' teams comprised the leading statutory health bodies leading and directing the HIA. Local community residents, both Dove Gardens residents and those from nearby neighbourhoods, were involved in the process. Members of the Local Assembly, Derry City Council and Local Strategic Partnerships were involved in the HIA also, comprising the representative and political element.

The Health Services in partnership: Cooperation and Working Together

CAWT operates on a partnership basis, by facilitating cross-border working on health and social care issues, and has established European connections in relation to the cross-border agenda. CAWT provides a forum which enables staff from health service organisations on both sides of the jurisdictional border to meet and work on cross-border health and social issues. At the time of writing, the CAWT partnership consists of six organisations: HSE in the Republic of Ireland and the Southern and Western Health and Social

Care Trusts in Northern Ireland. The Health and Social Care Board and the PHA in Northern Ireland are also CAWT partners (CAWT, 2014).

Northern Ireland Housing Executive (NIHE)
The NIHE is the regional housing authority. NIHE operated within its rights and duties to demolish and redesign more suitable accommodation in Dove Gardens estate in Derry. The Northern Ireland Housing Council was established by the Housing Executive Act (Northern Ireland) 1971. It is consulted by the NIHE and the Department of Social Development on issues pertaining to housing policy in Northern Ireland. The Housing Council consists of one representative of each of the twenty-six district councils in the region. By April 2015, this number of councils is planned to be reduced to eleven after the amalgamation process.

Due to the controversial nature of social housing in Northern Ireland, which was subject to charges of discrimination in service provision, particularly in the 1960s, changes had to be implemented to ensure greater fairness and transparency by the 1970s (Birrell and Hayes, 1999; McSheffrey, 2000; Tonge, 2005). Indeed, the Macrory Report (1970), which had been developed throughout the 1960s, faced new challenges and provisions by the time its provisions was legislated. In relation to housing matters, the contentious issue of housing was to be removed from local government to the more 'technocratic' and impartial NIHE, envisaged to allocate housing according to need in an unbiased and objective manner (Wilford *et al.*, 2007). NIHE today has an excellent track record in ensuring housing provision is based upon need, and so has developed a well-respected reputation and perception among the general public. Today NIHE continues to uphold its reputation as a fair, equitable and innovative public body. The interviews conducted for this overall study (phases I and II) strongly reiterated this message.

In Northern Ireland, whilst the provision of social housing remains in the hands of NIHE, the building programme of new houses and accommodation is completed by housing associations. In the last fifteen years the housing associations have been involved in the building of houses, whilst NIHE has not been involved since approximately 1996.

A respondent within NIHE clarified the role of NIHE and housing associations during phase II of data collection. A change in the role of the NIHE occurred five or six years ago, in that NIHE attained control of the managing process involved in the building of houses, which means that even though the body is not involved in the building, it has control over strategic decisions such as where the building can take place, the provision of grants to housing associations, and so on. These changes were implemented in-house, with the policy decision-making coming from the Department of Social Development on the government side, without any need for legislation. There has been no major legislation on housing in Northern Ireland for many years. At the time of writing there is discussion politically about the possibility of splitting the NIHE into two units, one being the landlord side (since the NIHE owns approximately 88,000 houses) and a strategic side (setting strategic direction on issues such as homelessness and so on). However this is still debate and conjecture; nothing has been finalised or decided in any way.

'Investing for Health' (IFH) Team (2002) (currently within the PHA)
Northern Ireland's health strategy, *Investing for Health* (2002), set out the Northern Executive's vision for population health improvement and for the reduction of health inequalities. *Investing for Health* (IFH) was founded on the principles of partnership working between the central government departments, local government, statutory, private sector, community and voluntary bodies and organisations. It was the strategy in place at the time the HIA was carried out, which strongly endorsed and called for HIAs to be conducted (DHSSPS, 2002).

Derry City Council
Derry City Council is the local government authority which includes the city area (including the Bogside community) within its remit. Due to the amalgamation of district councils in Northern Ireland as a result of the RPA, the new Derry City and Strabane District Council will be formed by 1 April 2015 (Derry City Council, 2014).

The Government Department of the Environment (DoE) is the statutory authority with responsibility over planning and development in Northern Ireland (Birrell and Hayes, 1999). However, a planning officer of the Planning Division of the DoE attends council meetings and answers questions put forward by local councillors; there exists formal consultative structures between the two authorities. From 1 April 2015, this system will change, resulting in councillors becoming the main decision-makers in planning (respondent from NILGA). In relation to the Dove Gardens HIA, the Planning Division (Strand Road, Derry) were invited to participate, as were planning officials within the council. Neither groups sent representatives to take part, although they were invited.

Apex Housing Group (North and West Housing Association)
The building for Dove Gardens was taken over by the housing association, namely Apex Housing Group. At the time of the Dove Gardens regeneration, there were thirty-nine such associations, and the policy target to meet housing need is for 1,500 to 2,500 units for social housing, in accordance with waiting lists. The changing nature of housing results in the need for close cooperation and working between the NIHE and housing associations which continues to this day.

Bogside and Brandywell Health Forum and Community Representation
The Brandywell and Bogside Health Forum (BBHF) was established in 1999 in order to assess the wellbeing and health of the community. It was set up initially as a working group. As a result of its work and the allocation of funding from the New Opportunities Fund (the Big Lottery Fund), the BBFH was granted assistance to establish a Healthy Living Centre initiative in the community (Lindsay, 2006). The Forum was locally born and developed 'as a response to the worsening situation in respect of ill health and health inequalities', which is commonly found in areas of social and economic deprivation (Doherty, 2006: 17). Other community groups in the area operate alongside the Forum, working on health and social issues raised by the community.

The BBFH has been in full operation since 2001. Its work spans over various areas, such as health promotion in the local primary schools, drug awareness programmes, older people's Monday Club, and the HIA on Dove Gardens has been cited as a large part of the Forum's overall work programme.

HIA methodology

A five-stage process of HIA was followed for this HIA. Screening guidelines, as developed by the Institute of Public Health were used, and the scoping checklist as developed by Ms. Erica Ison was used.

Both qualitative and quantitative methodologies were used in this HIA. A literature review was conducted on the evidence-base of housing and living conditions on human health. Four appraisal workshops were carried out in total. The purpose of these workshops was to marry what the residents said in the workshop about factors pertaining to the health impacts of the regeneration project, with evidence from the literature. A health profile was collated of the community, using local expertise, and information from the Northern Ireland Statistical and Research Agency (NISRA). It was the responsibility of the steering group to develop recommendations and to evaluate the impact of the HIA on the decision-making process (Glackin and Farrell, 2006).

HIA outcomes

In the case of this Dove Gardens prospective HIA, a positive outcome arising from the HIA was the amendment of the housing proposal in order 'to enhance the positive aspects and reduce or eliminate the negative impacts of redevelopment' (Glackin *et al.*, 2006). A number of recommendations were developed within the HIA which were to inform the decision-makers of the manner in which the regeneration scheme needed to be amended, in order to maximise the positive benefits and reduce the negative aspects. The results of the appraisal process were thirty-seven coded health impacts, from which thirty-five recommendations were produced. All of the recommendations are linked with one or more impact statements from the workshops. The areas within which recommendations were developed are indicated below.

For each sub-category within these recommendation areas, lead agencies were identified which would be responsible for implementing the recommendations:

The recommendations pertain to:

- Environment
- Homes and Housing
- Built Environment
- Sense of Community
- Service Provision
- Health Awareness
- Creating Local Jobs and Skills
- Partnerships. (Glackin and Farrell, 2006: 24)

As a result of the HIA process, a Dove Gardens resident group was established; there was an increase in stakeholder knowledge of their role in influencing health determinants; a working relationship between statutory, community and voluntary groups were established, which did not exist before; engaging local residents in the process has helped contribute to building sustainable community infrastructure; and the profile of HIA has been raised as a feasible instrument and approach to use in planning and community development. There was a possibility that NIHE would mainstream the use of HIA to all redevelopments and regeneration projects in Northern Ireland (Glackin and Farrell, 2006). However, this has not yet happened. Although NIHE does take account of social and health impacts as an integrated part of their work, the rising role of housing associations and the lesser role for NIHE means that even if NIHE were to promote HIAs to a greater extent, their role in housing has decreased.

Policy process for the Dove Gardens HIA

The steering group had representation from the key and primary decision-makers (the Northern Ireland Housing Executive and the North West Housing Association), which was vital to the development and dissemination of realistic recommendations that could be acted upon.

In order to monitor and evaluate the HIA, an Implementation Group was set up in order to 'oversee and influence the implementation of the recommendations of the HIA' (Glackin and Farrell, 2006: 30). This group comprised mainly of members of the steering group, which disbanded once the Implementation Group was established. The latter group will work closely with decision-makers to plan and organise for the delivery of the recommendations. To date all thirty-five recommendations have been included in the North West Housing Association design brief. It is the responsibility of the Implementation Group to ensure the recommendations are presented to all decision-making agencies and fora.

One of the key benefits of this HIA was the involvement of decision-makers at all stages of the HIA, from start to finish. The involvement of such an integral group has been identified in the literature as an enabler to the success of a HIA (Davenport *et al.*, 2006).

Part II: analysis

Interviews conducted with respondents for this HIA case were analysed and the findings from this analysis are presented in the following section. The conceptual lens, as outlined in Chapter 2, provides a framework for presenting the findings from the interviews. In this HIA case study, thirteen people were interviewed during phase I, from a variety of stakeholders who were involved in the HIA. For phase II, three people were interviewed.

'Institutions Matter': New Institutional Theory

Are institutions ready? The timing of HIA as a policy support tool

The timing of HIA as a policy support tool was raised during the interviews, with a view to gaining an insight into the perspective of those on the HIA steering group, which included both decision-makers of statutory bodies and those coming from a community perspective.

Except for two respondents, all those who were interviewed stated that yes, the time was right and had come for HIAs to be used in policy-making.

The two individuals who were interviewed from the NIHE organisation were more reticent about the timing of HIA utilisation. One respondent said that although the HIA was 'a labour of love', it would be after the monitoring and evaluation of the process after a number of years (after the residents have been re-housed in the new development) that the timing and appropriateness of the HIA could be assessed. From the same organisation, the area planner stated that 'it's too early for us yet to make that kind of assessment'. As far as these two respondents were concerned, they were going to 'wait and see the results' of the health and wellbeing of the residents in the regeneration project. Their attitude was more cautious in support of HIA, which may represent the organisational viewpoint of the instrument and approach in terms of its feasibility in the long term. The community worker from the Gasyard Centre was also cautious, stating that he would still 'reserve judgement until people are back in the new houses', even though this individual was adamant that the causal pathways between housing, health, education and employment that arose from the HIA findings are evidence that it should be used within policy with due timeliness and ease.

The other respondents stated that when HIAs are done correctly and in a rigorous manner they can be used in policy. The community worker from the Gasyard stated in response as to whether or not the time has come for policy-makers to use HIAs, 'yes, very beneficial, very clear lessons to be learnt, very clear causal links between health, education, employment and housing'. The individual from the Western Investing for Health (WIFH) team was in agreement with HIA timeliness, arguing that the policy direction of the central government in Belfast was 'forcing us to look at policy making and to make evidence based decisions'. The respondent from the BBHF agreed that the time had come for HIAs to be used in policy-making, as working in a multi-sectoral manner was the norm in policy-making and service delivery, from the community perspective, which the HIA approach advocated. The community and resident representative on the HIA agreed that the time had for its utilisation in policy, as it enhanced the regeneration process and ensured the 'residents are there, giving their opinion'. A respondent from CAWT believed that the time was right in the Dove Gardens case specifically, as there were high level decision-makers involved in the HIA, which made the process easier from a policy and evidence utilisation perspective. The respondent from the housing association agreed that the time had come for HIA to be used in policy, as it promoted community participation and joined-up working, which 'we're all supposed to do but never do so much in reality, but did with the HIA'.

Normative dimension: do institutions shape behaviour?

Those interviewed in this case were stakeholders in the HIA process, and were on the steering group as representatives of their relevant bodies, be it from statutory institutions (NIHE and North/West Housing Association), health services perspective (WIFH and SHSSB/CAWT) or the community perspective (Gasyard Community Centre, the BBFH, and the resident representative). At an institutional level, HIA process and policy process levels, a number of constraining factors upon behaviour were discussed in the interviews. Where the policy process level was concerned in this case study, it was policy formulation at the planning service level that was the constraining and problematic issue. Also, gathering local evidence and information for the HIA was a constraint in the conduct and thereafter use of the HIA. Beliefs and values also played a constraining role in this case study, in the use of the HIA and in the conduct of the process.

For this HIA, specific institutional bodies were openly named as acting as constraints to the process and subsequent use of the HIA findings in policy.

The housing association, planning services and roads services were identified by a respondent from the NIHE as constraints, their mindset being a constraining factor in the process and use of the HIA in policy or programme planning. These organisations were identified as lacking some commitment to the idea of HIA. The absence of such key stakeholders, and the lack of engagement of these players, was perceived as a constraint on the advance of the HIA use in policy (respondent from the BBHF). However as part of an interview during 2014, this respondent reflected that in the end, once the HIA was completed and the housing building was finished and the residents were back in their homes, the lack of engagement of key players did not have a lasting impact on the overall project. The lack of open and transparent sharing between the planning services and the NIHE was deemed as an institutional constraint on the maximum use of the HIA, and the absence of the planners from the process, particularly at the earliest stage of the HIA, was considered a negative factor in this HIA case study (NIHE respondent). Also, the tension between the community and statutory sectors was illustrated by one respondent from the BBHF:

> Some organisations, still, can retreat back into their silos very quickly when they're expected to contribute and make the project better. We've just to keep reminding people that this is a worthwhile project and worth going the extra mile, to make sure the problems are ameliorated.

On a related but separate issue regarding institutional constraints, and their impact on the HIA use, a NIHE respondent stated that it is vital to the HIA that the correct tier of decision-makers are accessed at a high level in their relative institutional setting, as 'one of the most important issues for us was, engaging with the correct partners, really it wasn't even engagement, and it was identification. Who are the partners that need to be engaged in this?' This individual stated that if the HIA was being conducted again, this engagement and identification of partners with a high degree of influence in their institutions would be a priority, as he felt those around the table did not have the breadth of knowledge and influence to maximise the use of the HIA in their relevant institutions. The issue of engagement of individuals with a high degree of influence was also raised by a respondent from CAWT, but in a more positive light. This individual stated that during the conduct of the HIA, the staff working on the rebuild (referring mainly to manual workers and builders) were not interested in the HIA: 'builders are just not concerned with community health and well being. There were constraints in the local management structures but the high level managers (from the NIHE) were on board and that's what matters.' The NIHE continues to have a strategic role in housing policy and direction in Northern Ireland at the time of writing.

At the level of the HIA, in terms of the conduct and process of it, a number of constraints were identified regarding the instrument. First, one respondent from the BBFH cited the fact that this HIA was the first conducted in the city as a constraining factor. Since it had never been conducted before, there was a certain amount of misunderstanding and wariness of the concept. This was reiterated by the community resident, who reflected that 'because it was a new thing for the NIHE and the North West housing association which is going to be in charge of the new housing, they didn't know what role the HIA should have'.

Second, the community resident on the HIA had a positive perspective of the process, and when asked about institutional constraints regarding this case, the individual referred to the fact that '(the HIA) might have pushed things to get things that we may not have got without it, they mightn't have given as much if we hadn't this on board. For definite the HIA helped push some issues onto the table'. This local resident identified the HIA process as enabling more resident preferences getting a priority in the housing redesign.

Third, the BBHF respondent said during the interview that a 'lack of knowledge and awareness of the HIA acted as barriers'. Indeed, the novelty of the instrument was considered a hindrance, as perceived from personal experience with HIA.

With regard to the policy process, some respondents referred to the planning process as a constraint in the use of HIA evidence to the maximum effect. At the end of the HIA, when the planning services were consulted, 'a long protracted process with planners' ensued and would have been alleviated if they had been present at earlier stages of the HIA, as observed by the community representative. The fact Derry City Council and the planning services were missing from the process, was a huge constraining factor in the successful conduct of the HIA and the appropriate use of its findings in policy thereafter, as reflected by the housing association respondent.

Value judgements and beliefs pertaining to the HIA concept were identified as institutional constraints during this phase of interviews.

One phrase was quoted and paraphrased by most of the interviewees during data collection (during phases I and II), which they believed illustrated succinctly the mindset of one of the key institutions that were involved in the regeneration and rebuilding process for Dove Gardens. An architect was quoted as saying: 'I build houses, I don't design communities.' A BBHF respondent reflected: 'but residents have to live there, so (this person) has to think beyond the drawing board.' For the purpose of this research the architect was unavailable for interview. Therefore, the statements and perceptions of those interviewed must be balanced against this proposition, and indeed a NIHE respondent was adamant that by the conclusion of the HIA process, this individual had changed beliefs around the need for community engagement in such regeneration projects, especially when the residents are displaced for a period of time before moving back into the new housing, as was the case for Dove Gardens residents.

Another issue that was brought up during the interviews (phase I) was the hindering role that knowledge and language played during the HIA process, and the need to overcome this obstacle, as identified by a NIHE respondent.

A member of the WIFH team stated that a constraining factor upon the use of HIAs is getting local evidence, community profiles and research on the locality, to feed into the HIA, which would then be envisaged for use in policy. This was deemed as an institutional constraint as the lack of research on the locality was deemed a barrier in ensuring appropriate services were planned into the future.

Political dimension: do politics matter?

This study investigated the influence of such a political dimension, by asking the interviewees to what extent politics were at play between the varying interests in the conduct of the HIA. Three issues arose from the responses to this question. The political dimension at a micro-level (individuals) and macro-level (institutions) was identified, and the use of the HIA tool to depoliticise the regeneration process was also found from the interviews.

Individuals: the gatekeepers to the institutions

With regards to politics at play, both in the conduct and aftermath of the HIA, some of the interview responses reflected that perhaps some individuals on the steering group were not the most appropriate individuals, meaning that some did not have the breadth of knowledge or worked at a high degree of decision-making influence required for the process. Indeed, a NIHE respondent said he would have 'been more selective with the people on the steering group'. The BBHF respondent stated that the HIA was targeted at the 'wrong people in organisations, the council didn't engage very well and that's probably because we targeted the HIA at the wrong people and they didn't see the benefit of it'.

On the other hand, there were key stakeholders who were not part of the HIA, and their involvement would have enabled the process to run smoother, as one respondent from the NIHE illustrated with regard to the planning services: 'I think it would have been constructive if the planning service had been there and could tell us the long term plan vision and given some sort of time frame.'

One respondent interpreted the 'politics' to refer to political parties and their role in the HIA. This individual stated that the political parties were invited to consult in the HIA but none came, which was no great loss according to a respondent in the NIHE, as 'the community were very capable of representing themselves'. This is an interesting observation and illustrates the degree of active citizenship and competence within the community groups.

Institutions: the gate and the building

In terms of the political dimension of the institutional influence upon HIA use for policy development, some interviewees identified tensions and politics between various institutions and organisations, such as between the NIHE and North/West Housing Association. A respondent from the NIHE stated that 'as the process went through there's a level of politics between ourselves and the housing association but you could have lifted that out, that hadn't anything to do with the HIA'. However, the tensions between the organisations impacted on the transfer of knowledge and information across institutional boundaries, and hindered the cohesive nature of housing design and planning that should have characterised the HIA. In addition to inter-institutional tensions, there were also tensions identified between different sectors, namely statutory and community, as highlighted by a member of the health services, who stated that there were 'definitely politics at play, big p and small p' between the NIHE and the community residents who were initially wary at becoming involved with the housing executive, due to antagonistic relations in previous times between the community and various statutory bodies.

A member of the WIFH team reflected that there was politics at play between different sectors and some members on the steering committee. This respondent illustrated that there were tensions between the planning services and everyone else involved in the HIA.

This tension and apprehension, which was interpreted as arising from the planning services, was identified as being related to the political culture within the organisation, as a respondent from the BBHF concluded. The ongoing reform of local government in NI, and the transfer of more planning functions to local authorities, may impact positively on the integration of planning services with endeavours such as HIA, specifically within the planned Community Planning aspect of the reform programme.

HIA: diluting the politics?

A theme that emerged from the interviews in response to the political dimension with the HIA, related to the dilution of politics in the housing project. The instrument and approach was deemed appropriate in depoliticising the process. A respondent from CAWT stated this point, that 'this was a new innovative way of working, so politics was counter balanced. During the scoping stage it's explicit about what will and won't be done, who will do it and won't, and it's explicit on the agenda'. The community representative stated that each of the stakeholders came to the HIA in good faith and with a shared interest in the regeneration of Dove Gardens, and so there were no politics at play from her perspective. The politics was diffused due to the stakeholders' common goal of a successful regeneration and rebuild process.

The role of value judgements in the HIA process

Three main points arose from the interviews regarding a questioning about the role of values and beliefs in the use of HIA knowledge for policy development. First, the institutional and organisational values played a role in the use and perception of the HIA. Second, the issue in evaluating the contribution to the HIA arose. Third, the need for balance between different types of evidence was raised, and the need to value all types.

Institutional and organisational values

A CAWT respondent stated very simply that values are everywhere and are undoubtedly present in the context of the HIA. A member of the WIFH team reflected that it was important on the steering committee to have a balance between professional values and communities values and interests, in order to ensure a balanced agenda. It was also important to ensure none of the institutions felt under attack, and so a balance within the statutory pool of people was also important. In addition, a BBHF respondent believed that organisational culture, and the values within such bodies, plays both a positive and negative role, as the following illustrates:

> I've no doubt that the organisational culture and the values from the organisations played both a positive and a negative role in the process. If you look at some of the statutory organisations they've always been at logger heads with communities, that's how they've existed, they've grown up separately and distinctly from the communities, some communities in Derry, and the HIA was seen as having to engage with communities. And that's seen as a threat. They're wary and sometimes hostile to it. We had to use a bit of guidance to around the hostility, we don't mind fighting but nowadays if you can find a way around fighting it's better.

How institutions view health inequalities was raised during the interviews also, and 'these inequalities in the area were profound and entrenched', as reflected by a respondent from the health services. The reduction of health inequalities is one of the founding pillars of the HIA concept. An understanding of the concept, health inequalities and the determinants of health is important for the successful process and outcome of HIAs.

Valuing contributions to the HIA

In terms of value judgements playing a role in the HIA process, issues were raised related to the improved values within the community regarding confidence and belief in its ability to articulate its views. A respondent from NIHE articulates this viewpoint succinctly in the following:

> Dialogue and community is marginalised, without this the tool was good to facilitate, HIA gave them greater input and they were allowed to increase voice

> and increase confidence … They would have a tree, garden, drive way, can have choice to buy car. Some things money can't buy and self-worth came from this.

The resident representative on the HIA reflected that the role of values and value judgements related solely to the values attributed to the community, and their input into the process. The HIA 'was about trying to make the best for the community for the people through the HIA … heightening the positive and lessening the negatives, which would be of value to the people that's what that was for, and I suppose with having residents on they were listening. They want what we wanted.'

Valuing the evidence balance

A respondent from CAWT reflected the there was a 'need for balance between research and community evidence, there's values about how both are viewed', which impacts on how evidence and information is perceived, collected and analysed within the context of a HIA. The evidence on health impacts then goes on to be used, it is hoped, within the institutions that decide on policy, and their value judgements on different types of evidence also plays an important role in the assimilation of types of knowledge and evidence in policy-making.

Knowledge use for policy development

Each respondent was asked to what extent, as far as they knew, was the HIA used in policy and how useful was the HIA.

Policy-making process

In terms of HIA use for policy development, and the degree to which it was used in policy and in other ways, the respondents perceived that it was used within the policy-making processes. An enabling factor was identified by the team member of the WIFH, who stated that with regard to the use of the HIA, 'timing is important, getting into the policy process early enough' is deemed the most successful way of evidence and knowledge being used. Also, another enabling factor was the involvement of high-level decision-makers in the HIA, which was the case with this Dove Gardens project. The recommendations were used at policy level, 'especially health and policy level, which were addressed at policy level by the NIHE and taken on by the health services', as stated by a BBHF respondent. Indeed, the same individual went on to say that 'everyone talks about consulting communities but few methods or approaches actually do it properly, and the HIA gives a good basis for that, engagement, and for trying out new ideas. I think it's a good basis for policy development'.

A respondent from CAWT reflected that it is 'useful in getting health on the agenda of policy makers, it's a must. HIA is one way of getting health on the agenda of policy makers from outside the health sector'. As illustrated here, HIA is identified as an appropriate instrument in raising health awareness of policies, projects and programmes with policy-makers.

Institutional utilisation

In terms of the institutionalisation of HIA, there was work being done at the strategic level of the NIHE to mainstream the tool, so that it would be conducted on all urban regeneration projects, and for all developments in the coming years, as was stated in the interviews with respondents from CAWT and NIHE. However, by 2014, this mainstreaming had not happened, and it remains to be seen if it could be embedded within the implementation of local government reform, which by April 2015 will result in more planning and regeneration functions being transferred to local authorities.

Spatial planning services

In every interview, without exception, the planning services were mentioned. However, the responses in this section must take into account that a respondent from the planning services, although approached, was not available for interview. The lack of involvement of this stakeholder in an urban regeneration project was viewed as a serious failing in the process and framework of action of the HIA. A CAWT respondent said that 'if planners were involved, it's better. Planners think in terms of exits and entrances of the building, not in terms of what goes on inside'. A BBHF respondent reiterated the sentiment of this statement, explaining that 'I don't think it (HIA) has impacted on the planning service, which is a major issue … At city level I'd say it hasn't impacted at all'. These are two statements were made in response to this question regarding the use of the HIA by the end of the process. However, throughout the entire round of interviews, the identification of the absence of the planning services and the manner in which this was a barrier in the full use of the HIA was relayed by all respondents. This indicates the importance the planning services role was regarded, and the important value placed on their input into the process of HIAs.

HIA

In terms of the further use of the HIA on the Dove Gardens estate, respondents from NIHE stated that monitoring and evaluation of the process was required so as to establish the health gain and health outcomes that the community experience three years after they have moved back into the new housing. This focus upon health gain as an appraisal indicator for the effectiveness of HIA is difficult to measure, as has been outlined in the research rationale of the European study on HIA effectiveness in decision-making processes across the continent, completed by Wismar *et al.* (2007). However, this was an important facet to the outcome measurement for the NIHE, as the greater the increase in community gain post-redevelopment, the greater the credibility the organisation will attribute to HIA. A review of the HIA was conducted by Bonner (2011) and will be discussed in greater detail below.

A respondent from the NIHE also stated that until the instrument is mainstreamed and legislated it would continue to be used on an ad-hoc basis, and not in a systematic manner. However, there were numerous impacts that the HIA had upon the rebuild, which 'is all specifically a consequence of the HIA'.

An example of this was in relation to educational space in the bedrooms of the new housing. The residents recommended that there be space for study desks in each of the bedrooms, so that children 'would not compete with the television when doing their homework' (CAWT respondent). The new development now has study space for children, which is hoped to impact on those who attend third level education in the long run, as just 1 per cent of the population attended third level education (Bonner, 2007).

Work practices

A respondent from CAWT, when reflecting on the HIA process, was adamant that many intangible benefits and outcomes arose from the HIA, namely the positive influence the HIA had on people in their work practice and intersectoral partnership working.

Recommendations

According to the resident representative, who is also a member of the Local Implementation Group (which came into existence after the HIA finished carrying out the recommendations of the process) and a member of the Dove Gardens Design Team, 'a lot of the recommendations have been used' for the redesign process.

Part III: update on the Dove Gardens HIA

A review of the Dove Gardens HIA was carried out by the PHA in 2011 (Bonner, 2011). Out of the total of thirty-seven impact statements and recommendations, twenty-nine (78 per cent) were fully achieved, seven (19 per cent) partly achieved and one (3 per cent) had yet to be determined (Bonner, 2011). Some recommendations that were formulated within the HIA were already part of the procedures of the NIHE and housing associations. The HIA process itself, and the added value that it brought to the regeneration design and implementation and to the local community and people, is the aspect of the project that had a lasting effect, in addition to the implementation of the specific recommendations.

As part of the review of the impact of the Dove Gardens HIA (Bonner, 2011), a door-to-door survey was conducted with the sixty-three dwelling residents. This survey revealed highly positive evaluations on the part of the residents of the former Dove Gardens housing and the new redevelopment. Ninety-five per cent stated that they were proud of Dove Gardens, which is triple the satisfaction rating recorded since before the redevelopment started. Those who said they loved living on the estate more than doubled to 90 per cent. Seventy-eight per cent revealed they were optimistic for the future, a significant increase on the 20 per cent rating prior to the redevelopment. The improvement in the payment for fuel in the new redevelopment was noted as a significant success of the project, as fuel poverty was a major problem in the former development. Due to solar panels and more efficient heating systems in the buildings, the residents are now paying less for their heating, a very positive outcome for the redevelopment, as stated by one resident who claims to save £25 per week now in the new development: 'Better heating, lovely, solar panel brilliant' (Bonner, 2011: 18). For those at greater risk of fuel poverty (lone parents and older people), the savings of more than £20 per week, as reported by residents, means that those groups in particular benefited 'exceptionally well' from the redevelopment (Bonner, 2011: 19). This addresses a finding based on research that between Northern Ireland and the Republic of Ireland, lone parents and older people are the most vulnerable groups at risk of fuel poverty (McAvoy, 2007). Clearly the redevelopment had been a success on many counts. One community resident correlated the conduct of the HIA on the redevelopment proposal as having a positive impact on the resulting redevelopment:

> The new build in Dove Gardens went beyond anything anyone anticipated and as a resident who was involved from the beginning of this process I believe we owe a lot of our success to the HIA that was carried out in Dove Gardens. (Bonner, 2011: 60)

However, the success of the HIA did not result in other HIAs on housing projects being conducted in the area or jurisdiction in the wake of the Dove Gardens redevelopment. The momentum for HIA was not seized by stakeholders in the way that was hoped. With the restructuring of the health services, particularly the creation of the PHA in 2009, and the upcoming restructuring of local authorities (which will involve a transfer of planning and regeneration functions to local authorities), there is much upheaval as to the work being done which may have impacted and will impact on HIAs being conducted, in both positive and negative ways. A respondent from the PHA reflected that the changes in personnel as part of the creation of the PHA resulted in much loss of expertise, experience and enthusiasm for HIA when employees were relocated to different offices. Regarding the role of NIHE in mainstreaming HIA more as part of their operations, it was noted by a respondent from Belfast Health City partnership that the NIHE in particular prioritises a consideration of social and health impacts in its planning policies, which may mean that standalone HIAs are not always necessary. Also, without HIA being placed on a legislative footing, it is difficult for individuals to take up the instrument voluntarily. Even with the best will and intention in the world, if individuals do not have HIA specified as part of their job description and are over-burdened with other tasks, it is difficult then for an HIA to be initiated and followed through. As one respondent from the Chartered Institute of Environmental Health Northern Ireland succinctly expressed: 'if HIA is optional, then it will stay optional.' However, with the current WHO designation of Healthy City status for Derry City Council and the expertise in HIA being garnered within the council at the moment, this illustrates the potential home for HIA in the area in the future. Strabane District Council was involved in an HIA on a community allotment proposal (Institute of Public Health in Ireland, 2013) and its experience with the process also bodes well for the continued use of the instrument once Derry and Strabane councils amalgamate from April 2015.

Lessons learned: community participation and HIA

As in Chapter 4, the HIAs explored in this chapter illustrate the way that the instrument can facilitate greater intersectoral partnership and can inform a statutory housing programme (TAP) and an urban regeneration project. The way in which the two HIAs in this chapter informed local policies and plans differed. For the TAP, the HIA had many benefits, as it brought various stakeholders together to work on a health-focused assessment project, resulted in health evidence that has been at least referred to in the subsequent policy programmes, and the HIA ensured peer researchers in the community were trained, enabling them to work on future health research projects. However, the entrenched issues of opposing views and concerns were palpable and impacted on the HIA before it had even begun. This calls into question whether HIA is suitable for such a highly sensitive topic area, as the expectations it can raise may not be reached according to all stakeholders involved. This can have damaging long-term effects for future intersectoral work. At least, expectations need to be raised and discussed at the beginning of a project. In the Dove Gardens redevelopment housing project, the HIA clearly influenced the redesign of the project plan and ensured the community voice was recognised and shaped (as reflected by the community itself) the design of the new housing, as well as the process of this redesign. Despite missing some partners in the process (notably the spatial planning services), the HIA appears to have been used instrumentally in the redevelopment plan. It is unfortunate that the HIA did not inspire a spate of HIAs on further housing projects. However this may also have been due to the fact that some organisations such as NIHE already systematically consider social and health impacts of their policies and plans. Time will tell if HIA will be integrated more into policy development processes after the implementation of local government by April 2015 (once the local government reform programme is implemented). This reform will involve measures such as the transfer of relevant functions for HIA to the local authorities (regeneration and planning) and the initiation of the Community Planning aspect of reform.

The expectations of the community within the process of an HIA is a key issue for those leading the project to be mindful of, especially if the project starts off with such expressed expectations, some of which may be unrealistic. Such high hopes are not an inherently bad thing; however they can be easily dashed if others around the HIA table are unable or unwilling to deliver on the expected actions and to the extent that has been hoped. This can seriously damage future intersectoral partnership working.

The input and participation of the community groups in both HIAs was a positive development. The following illustrates this point, as outlined by one resident and former HIA steering group member in the Dove Gardens HIA:

> The community spirit in Dove Gardens is at an all time high and it is something I haven't felt since I was a child myself, thanks to our shared experiences, the HIA team and Apex Housing, Dove Gardens is one of the best places in Derry to live and it is with immense pride now that we welcome people into our area and there is never any shortage of people as the Gasyard Centre celebrates every social event in the calendar, our children are catered for in a way I have never seen before from parades to street parties and we the adults are not left out either with fitness and education courses run on a daily basis. (Bonner, 2011: 60)

Conclusion

As demonstrated from the two HIAs explored in this chapter, the input of the community and lay knowledge to the HIA, and subsequently to the policy-making processes, was integral not only to the overall success of the proposed plan, project or policy (such as Traveller accommodation policy or urban housing redesign) but also to the acceptability of state policies, programmes and plans by those people on the receiving side. However the input of community knowledge is also a contentious issue as especially indicated by the TAP HIA. In both HIAs evidence from the process was used to inform the housing programmes, varying in their degrees of use. Both HIAs illustrate how this instrument and approach is sometimes used to dilute the politics, either to dilute the political nature and controversy of the topic (such as Traveller accommodation) or cross-institutional politics such as with the Dove Gardens HIA and the history of housing politics in the city. In the HIA on the TAP, the statutory body that was expected to use the HIA the most, by implementing it as part of future housing initiatives and TAPs, was by no means the main instigator or leader on the HIA. This then had significant implications in terms of the user/owner dynamic in the use of HIA knowledge for policy development. As one respondent stated in the HIA on the TAP, 'all politics is local in Donegal', and absolutely nothing could be done subsequently regarding Traveller accommodation in the county without the agreement and support of the council's elected members.

The following chapter will examine the four HIAs together, exploring the similarities and differences of their use in policy development, in direct and indirect ways, through the conceptual lens as outlined in Chapter 2. It will also highlight some key conclusions and recommendations based on this book's research.

6

Making a difference

Informing policy development

Four HIAs were explored as to their use for policy development as part of a qualitative longitudinal study. This final chapter seeks to reflect on the conceptual lens that was used to examine the influences on the use of the HIAs for policy development, and the extent of their use. Additionally, common conclusions based on the practical conduct of HIAs are discussed. Reflections on the future of HIA are also discussed in this chapter.

HIA for policy development: a conceptual lens

A conceptual lens drawing on relevant theories was used to explore the HIA instrument and how it could inform policy development. More often than not, knowledge and evidence intended for policy development will be used in some way, and it is this degree of use that is being captured in the conceptual lens. The conceptual lens drew from three main schools of literature and thought (Chapters 2 and 3):

1. Institutional theory (incorporating HIA literature on the political dimension).
2. Discourse analysis, IA literature and the role of value judgements.
3. Policy analysis and knowledge utilisation.

The conceptual lens was devised in a very pragmatic way so as to explore the influences on HIA use for policy development, a novel area of study and unique in the context of the jurisdictions on the island of Ireland. The lens was founded on a premise that individuals are influenced by factors beyond their control, and often beyond their awareness, which could impact on the way that HIA processes and outcomes can inform policy development.

The following includes an examination of the micro (individual actors and their value judgements) and macro (institutional structures and the associated normative and political dimensions) levels of analysis. This is in line with the following overarching research question: *how* and *why* do the overarching structures and underlying values influence the use of HIAs in policy?

The following sections illustrate the application of the conceptual lens across the four HIAs and assesses the suitability of the chosen theories and schools of literature so as to answer the research questions. For greater ease of description, the HIAs are referred to in relation to their geographical location. A summary of the findings of the HIAs is outlined also.

HIAs in the RoI and NI

Four HIAs were explored in this book, two from the RoI and two from NI. The HIAs were conducted in the areas of the physical environment (air quality and traffic and transport) and housing. The HIA on traffic and transport in Ballyfermot, Dublin, was used to inform traffic-calming measures in the community and a number of health promotion activities in the area. The HIA on the Draft Air Quality Action Plan in Belfast was used to inform the statutory action plan and to ensure the community voice was included in the final outcome. The HIA conducted on the TAP in Donegal was an oppositional case out of the four HIAs. It was initiated in order primarily to amend and inform the implementation of the statutory programme in the county. It was used to inform the programme, however the extent of this usage is subject to debate. The HIA on the social housing estate Dove Gardens in Derry/Londonderry informed the redesign of the project and also ensured that the affected resident community had a meaningful voice in the process. The following sections examine how the conceptual lens assessed the influences on the use of the HIAs for policy development, and the extent of this use.

New Institutional Theory

How do institutional structures influence HIA use in policy?
New Institutional Theory was chosen to explain the influence of overarching structures that have the potential to shape individual behaviour and action, or non-action (Immergut, 1992; March and Olsen, 1984; 2005; Peters, 1999). The degree of convergence and divergence in the themes that arose from the interviews will be used to illustrate the practicability of this theory to explain the phenomena of influence on HIA use in policy-making.

In response to the question of institutional constraints and these impacts upon individual behaviour and the way in which HIA use for policy development may be affected, there was a mix of convergence and divergence of themes or patterns that arose from the interviews. The findings presented here all arose from the interview data itself. All HIAs converged on the categories of institutions as an influence upon behaviour at a macro-level, and the HIA process and the policy process as influences on the lower micro-level. This convergence or agreement indicates the degree of institutional influences, and the norms that such institutional structure exudes as influences, across the cases despite the difference in case study settings, topics and geopolitical locations.

'Evidence' arose in the two Northern Ireland cases, Belfast and Derry/Londonderry. Both HIAs highlighted the issue of accessing local evidence for policy-aiding mechanisms. A lack of local evidence and community profiles constrains the HIA process and the subsequent use of the knowledge that comes from this process for policy development, as well as delaying the HIA as local evidence may have to be gathered as part of the IA methodology.

In both the Derry/Londonderry and Donegal cases the influence of values, beliefs and ideas acted as institutional constraints. In the former HIA, an entrenched attitude of a senior architect contributed to constrained statutory engagement in the HIA process. This was in large part attributed to the individual's own beliefs that it was the job of architects to 'build houses, but not [to] design communities'. In the Donegal HIA, ideas were deemed constraints as the subjective values and beliefs people held about the topic of Traveller accommodation (both sides of opinion) overtook the objective worthiness of the evidence that came from the HIA (Davenport *et al.*, 2006).

In divergence, patterns arose from the cases that were specific to each the individual HIA. In the Donegal HIA, the topic of Traveller policy was itself a constraint and the institutional prejudices and attitudes acted as barriers to the willing engagement in the HIA and in its aftermath. In the Derry/Londonderry HIA, the absence of the planning services was highlighted as a key constraint on the activity of other stakeholders around the table, as this is a vital partner missing from the process, although in phase II of the study, the absence of this partner did not have a longer-term impact on the use of HIA for the development. The lack of community resources and infrastructure in the Belfast HIA was identified as a constraint upon behaviour of the statutory stakeholders, and added time delays in engaging with the community sector for the HIA.

Political dimension

Previous academic research, investigating the use of HIAs in policy-making, has established the influence of the political context upon HIA evidence utilisation (Bekker, 2007). The direct and indirect influence of the political environment, and actor's preferences in policy-making, are important considerations when investigating influences on HIA use (Bekker *et al.*, 2005; Elliott and Francis, 2005; Putters, 2005).

All four HIAs assessed in this study acknowledged the influence of the individuals who were the micro-level gatekeepers to the institutions being investigated, and the influence of the institutions themselves as the 'gates and buildings'. This thematic agreement illustrates the feasibility of the political dimension as an explanation of the influences on HIA use, the acknowledgement of the influence of the political environment and actor's preference, and how the institution may affect and shape the behaviour of individuals.

Politics with a small 'p' (institutional politics) was identified as an influence upon individual behaviour in the Donegal and Ballyfermot HIAs, as has been identified in previous research (Bekker *et al.*, 2004; Elliott and Francis, 2005). The HIA process was viewed as an advocacy tool in the Belfast and Donegal HIAs; as a tool which would be used to endorse particular standpoints, and therefore was not neutral or objective (Kemm and Parry, 2004). The area of Traveller work and policy, and the vested interests at play amongst all stakeholders, was highlighted as part of the political dimension. In the Derry/Londonderry HIA respondents viewed the instrument as a mechanism that would dilute the politics of urban regeneration amongst the statutory stakeholders, and within their institutional interests and structures.

A clash of opinions occurred regarding which evidence was deemed correct in the area of transport, traffic and air quality in the Ballyfermot case. The disagreement that exists between expert and lay evidence was highlighted in this HIA under study.

In the Belfast HIA the expectations of it were not managed appropriately. Priorities and expectations of the process should have been established at the beginning of the endeavour, so as to avoid unmet expectations and disappointment in the HIA process. This point was concluded from the European evaluation of HIA effectiveness in policy (Wismar *et al.*, 2007). This issue of expectations of the process was also the case in the Donegal HIA.

The need for HIA legislative recognition and institutional embeddedness was highlighted in the Donegal HIA, as has been pointed out in previous research (Banken, 2001; Bekker *et al.*, 2004; Davenport *et al.*, 2006; Wismar *et al.*, 2007; O'Mullane, 2013), and was also raised during phase II of the study, by respondents from the Institute of Public Health, HSE, Chartered Institute of Environmental Health Northern Ireland and PHA.

Value judgements and the IA paradigm

How do value judgements influence HIA use for policy development?

It is important to take account of the role that value judgements play in policymaking. Such judgements relate to the perception of what a 'good' decision is over another group's perception or understanding, and the two may have diverging points of view. In order to avoid rationalising the policy process to any idealistic extreme, the role that values play in the consideration of HIAs in policy is an integral aspect of this study. It is important to note that such value judgements are context-dependent and institutionally influenced, meaning that individuals are influenced by the setting of their work and the values implied within that setting.

The WHO Gothenburg Consensus paper (1999), the most cited document in HIA literature, highlights the pertinence of values underlying the processes, institutions and actors that HIAs are attempting to influence. The WHO paper emphasises the need to consider the influence of values upon decision-making processes and the need to take them into account when establishing the influence that HIAs can have upon such processes (ECPH, 1999).

Value judgements, and the role that values play in the use of HIAs for policy-making, were identified in this study. Institutional and organisational values were highlighted in the Belfast and Derry/Londonderry HIAs, as the respondents were adamant that value judgements played a role in the use, or non-use, of the HIA in policy development, and indeed during the HIA process. What is considered good evidence for policy, and what is cast aside, was influenced by the institutional and organisational value judgements. Institutional complexity, negative attitudes towards the process, and the need to persuade institutions and individuals (Majone, 1989) of the benefits of HIAs and the knowledge coming from the process, were raised in the Ballyfermot HIA. Respondents in the Ballyfermot HIA stated that HIAs must be legislated for if they are to be mainstreamed and not conducted on an ad-hoc or opportunistic basis only, which has been identified in previous research (Wismar *et al.*, 2007).

Valuing the evidence balance between lay knowledge and expert knowledge was highlighted in the Derry/Londonderry HIA, which was also raised in the Belfast HIA in relation to the values placed upon the contributions to the process.

Values attributed to the conceptualisation of health, in a more holistic sense, impacted on the use of HIA knowledge, as the Donegal and Belfast HIAs indicated. The contributions and involvement of the community sector in the HIA (Ballyfermot) and the attitudes towards a particular community group, the Travellers (Donegal), illustrated the importance that value judgements play in all aspects of the HIA process, and not only in relation to the utilisation of knowledge for policy-making.

Values implicit in the policy process and those of the stakeholders, who are envisaged to use the HIA knowledge, was a determining factor in the Belfast HIA, as was the issue of policy entrepreneurs and the impact that innovative individuals across the various institutional boundaries had on the use of HIAs for policy.

A miscommunication of values and especially of expectations in the Donegal HIA illustrates the need for better clarity at the commencement of the HIA process, as previous research has highlighted (Wismar *et al.*, 2007).

The hypothesised influences (overarching institutional and underlying values) on the use of the HIAs for policy development in the conceptual lens are applicable in this study, as illustrated in the above. The following section outlines the extent of use of HIAs for policy development.

Were the HIAs used in policy? The dimensions of direct and indirect use for policy development

This section illustrates the extent of the use of the four HIAs for policy development, using the conceptual lens outlined in Chapter 2.

Policy analysis and utilisation theories

Why is the degree of use, both direct and indirect, varied in different contexts?

The hypothesised outcome, which in this case is the extent to which HIAs are used for policy development, will be assessed in terms of the degree of knowledge utilisation, as indicated in Table 6.1. Policy analysis and knowledge utilisation theories informed the construction of this hypothesised outcome from each HIA case and the direct and indirect utilisation indicators (Chapter 2).

The work of Janowitz (1970), who recognised the potential for conceptual utilisation of knowledge over time, labelled this process as 'enlightenment'. The consideration of politics underlying the use of knowledge and the evaluation of policy rejects the rationalistic approach to evaluation, and recognises the degree of policy learning that can occur in the policy processes; direct use of knowledge is no longer the only form of utilisation that is recognised, given the political nature of using knowledge in policy (Patton, 1997; Sanderson, 2002; Rossi *et al.*, 2004).

This section of the chapter will examine each HIA for the three degrees of utilisation of HIA knowledge (as outlined also in Chapter 2), taking account of the influences on use (institutional and value judgements). First, the convergence of themes that were found indicates contingent generalisations that can be made across the cases regarding use for policy development.

By the end of the longitudinal study, the recommendations from the four HIAs under study (called suggestions in the Belfast case) were used *instrumentally (directly)* in policy formulation. At the time of phase I of the study, it was concluded that the HIA in the Donegal case was not used instrumentally (directly), neither to inform present-day policy, nor improve the TAP retrospectively. However during phase II it was found that the HIA was incorporated into the two subsequent TAPs and is, at least, referred to as being a source of evidence on the part of the local authority, which is the institution which formulates the TAP in consultation with stakeholders. Since the definition used for instrumental use of the HIA for policy development is 'the documented and specific use of knowledge' (Rossi *et al.*, 2004: 411), it must be concluded that it was indeed instrumentally (directly) used. However, this is concluded with reticence as the stakeholders involved held such polar opposite views as to what constituted the implementation of the HIA within the TAPs, that this conclusion will be contingent on a full-scale evaluation of the HIA implementation in practice taking place.

The policy-making process, and policy environment in the case of Ballyfermot, was informed directly by the findings of the HIA and the knowledge was used to inform policy. However, a full utilisation of all recommendations was not found in all cases, with greater instrumental utilisation evident in Belfast and Derry, to a lesser degree in Ballyfermot, and the Donegal case displaying the least instrumental utilisation of the HIA.

In all cases, the HIA process highlighted the degree to which the findings of the process would be used. The HIA indicated the level of factionalised power across the various institutions in the Belfast case which acts as an inhibitor to the use of knowledge in the long run, in addition to the local government reform process being a constraint, at least until 1 April 2015; in the Ballyfermot case the future of the HIA was guaranteed at least for a time after its conclusion through the creation of the Impact Group. Although this has since dissolved, the HIA process has been cited as directly influencing the initiation of various initiatives in the area, as confirmed by a respondent from DCC (Community and Social Development Department) in phase II of the study. The HIA process in Derry/Londonderry highlighted the benefits of cross-sectoral collaboration and the policy learning and enlightenment that can come from such processes. The HIA has informed the redevelopment as was highlighted in its review (Bonner, 2011), and although the impact it has had on health gain has not yet been specifically established, it is clear that the redevelopment, informed by the HIA, has reduced fuel poverty in the area. The HIA process in the Donegal case highlighted the need for political will and genuine statutory stakeholder commitment to the project for the long term.

In terms of *conceptual (indirect) utilisation*, defined as 'the use of knowledge to influence thinking about issues in a general way' whereby the HIA would be used in a general way to inform policy indirectly, all cases fit into this categorisation (Rossi *et al.*, 2004: 411).

Respondents in the Ballyfermot case indicated the manner in which the HIA would 'drip into policy, not (be) an explosive contribution to policy but may inform it indirectly' (respondent from the Institute of Public Health). This point was reiterated by another respondent from DCC in the case also. The HIA was identified as contributing findings on traffic and transport that the community could use into the future. The findings were also used to inform health promotion and health services activities in the vicinity, as well as initiatives such as the Cold Weather Response Initiative, which indicates the indirect utilisation of HIA knowledge.

Respondents in the Donegal case also highlighted the fact that although the HIA may not be immediately used in policy, it may be a 'brick in the wall towards something more substantial. It started as a process and may show results down the road' (HIA researcher). This was also raised by other respondents in the case, however the polarisation of attitudes towards Traveller accommodation between the stakeholders in this case acts more as a barrier to the use of HIA findings, rather than any implicit failing of the HIA in this case.

Respondents in the Belfast case stated that in addition to the HIA informing the action plan concurrently, it also was being used in policy formulation within the Environmental Health section of BCC, and would be used to inform the planning review as led by the planning services, providing in particular the community perspective for the city's Masterplan.

Respondents in the Derry/Londonderry case stated that alongside the HIA being used instrumentally to inform the redesign and regeneration of the Dove Gardens estate, it was used by the local health services and the community health forum (BBHF) to provide adequately tailored local community health services.

In terms of *persuasive (indirect) utilisation*, defined as the use of knowledge 'to either support or refute political positions – in other words, to defend or attack the status quo', whereby the HIA will be used to endorse a particular standpoint, two of the cases can be categorised in this grouping (Rossi *et al.*, 2004: 411).

Respondents in the Belfast HIA, in particular those on the management team, stated that the HIA was used as another means of facilitating collaboration and partnership between the statutory stakeholders. Entrenched attitudes, institutional dormancy and immovable institutional standpoints had brought the formulation of the Draft Air Quality Action Plan almost to a standstill as was concluded from phase I of the study. It was at this point the HIA was introduced, to facilitate collaboration and to inform stakeholders of the wider determinants of health, which was not considered by the majority of non-health sector statutory stakeholders. In this case, the HIA was used as an advocacy tool, endorsing a particular direction and with underlying expectations for improving collaborative mechanisms. The way that the HIA was used as an implicitly (institutionally) political means to a political end was raised by respondents in phase I of the study. Such immovable institutional standpoints do not seem to be present for the development of the upcoming Air Quality Action Plan, and an HIA is not planned to be conducted on this upcoming plan, as it was for the previous one.

Respondents in the Donegal HIA explained how the HIA was introduced as a mechanism that could 'cut through politics' (respondent from the Donegal Traveller Group) and could facilitate better working relations between the county council and the Donegal Traveller Project in particular. A history of tension was characteristic of the topic in the area, and the HIA was expected to reduce these polarised attitudes, or at least keep them outside the HIA process.

Table 6.1 The degree of use of the HIAs for policy development

Degree of utilisation	*Instrumental (direct)*	*Conceptual (indirect)*	*Persuasive (indirect)*
Ballyfermot	√	√	/
Donegal	√	√	√
Belfast	√	√	√
Derry	√	√	√

Instrumental: Ballyfermot, Belfast, Derry, Donegal.
Conceptual: Ballyfermot, Donegal, Belfast, Derry.
Persuasive: Donegal, Belfast, Derry.

Respondents in the Derry/Londonderry case also viewed the HIA tool as a means of diluting the politics of housing, as this subject is a historically controversial one, and the HIA mechanism was viewed as a means of neutralising any friction in the debate on the urban regeneration project. It was also a means of including the policy receivers (local resident community) in the process, who had been historically excluded from the processes in Derry, which had devastating effects, which are still in the communal memory of the area.

Table 6.1 indicates the degree of applicability the utilisation typology has for this research. All HIAs fit into each of the three categories, whilst Ballyfermot is applied to instrumental and conceptual use.

Overall, the theories of knowledge utilisation and policy analysis have informed an appropriate and feasible utilisation measure for policy. There is variance in the applicability across the cases, which can be explained by the institutional and value judgements that impacted upon HIA use for policy development in this study.

Longitudinal HIA study: phase I (2007/8) and phase II (2013/14)

This book is based on a qualitative longitudinal study which included two phases of research taking place in sequential time periods to examine the development or progress of increased use of the HIA evidence over a longer period of time. A total of fifty-eight interviews took place.

Respondents in phase II of the study were asked if they believed, based on experience, that the conduct and development of HIA has been negatively impacted by the economic recession which hit both jurisdictions since the four HIAs were conducted. In relation to HIA, a clear majority of respondents did not believe the economic recession impacted on HIA development. A greater influence on the practice of HIA, has been the restructuring of the health services and local government. These changes have been happening to varying degrees in both jurisdictions. Respondents from the Institute of Public Health stated that based on actual numbers of HIAs, there were more conducted post-2008 than between 2001 and 2008 (across both jurisdictions). Respondents did note that perhaps there was extra money and resources 'floating around' in 2008 and 2009, and perhaps now that austerity measures are in place, a decline in HIA numbers may be observed from 2013 onwards. However this remains to be seen. In Northern Ireland, the adoption of the more pragmatic HIA approach was driven primarily to fit HIA for purpose, and second to make the process more efficient. For the upcoming Air Quality Action Plan, local authority respondents stated that a HIA approach would be adopted rather than a comprehensive HIA, as with the previous plan. Reasons cited for this were based on government resourcing cutbacks and a preference for a HIA approach to assessing the plan for health impacts rather than a full-scale process. In final conclusion, it seems that the economic recession has not had a greatly negative impact on the conduct and development of HIAs, and the more flexible and pragmatic approach to HIA conduct is more related to it being tailored for specific contexts rather than in order to save money and resourcing.

The public health strategies that have been released in the RoI (2013, *Healthy Ireland*) and in NI (2014, *Making Life Better*) advocate for HIA in a different way compared to the strategies of 2001 (RoI) and 2002 (NI). Perhaps the way that HIA is being promoted in the most recent strategies is based on a more realistic vision of the instrument, which can be used as part of another IA (SIA in the RoI) or as an instrument to advance the HiAP agenda (NI). Time will reveal if the vision for HIA in the public health strategies will ensure greater assessment of health impacts of projects, programmes and policies. Both phases of the study highlighted the necessity of legislative recognition of HIA, as without this vital step, the conduct and sustainability of the instrument and approach is unsure and dependent on enthusiastic people to keep the practice alive within their organisations. In the Derry/Londonderry HIA under study, it was concluded by the end of phase I that although it would have been beneficial overall to the process if the planning services were involved in the HIA when it was conducted, by the time the housing was built, the impact of their absence had less impact than previously envisaged by respondents in phase I. This illustrates that the HIA process can have a positive impact with some partners missing from the process.

Policy rhetoric and reality: HIA in the RoI and NI

The discussion in Chapter 2 regarding the conceptual roots of HIA illustrated the varied influences on the development of HIA, including the policy environment. Chapter 3 illustrated the systems in place at a local level and the reform processes in both jurisdictions, which will have an impact on the conduct of the HIA instrument and the HiAP approach generally. The public health strategies released in both jurisdictions that refer to HIA have been discussed, in terms of the policy context. The 'translation gap' that exists between the statements in policy documents and strategies, and the implementation of clauses on the ground, is evident in relation to HIA (Kearns and Pursell, 2011). The conceptual lens used and applied to the four HIAs in this book shows us one way to bridge this gap, by being mindful of the influences on HIA use in policy development, and the extent that HIA knowledge can be used for policy development. The findings of this lens' application to the HIAs are generalisable across HIA in general and in a variety of country contexts. The learning from this study may be translated and used in other jurisdictions, accounting for specificities of the HIAs under study from both jurisdictions.

HIA in practice

A key change that has happened in NI and to some extent in the RoI is the evolution of HIA in practice. It has developed from a time of conducting traditional full-scale comprehensive HIAs towards a situation whereby a more pragmatic approach to using a flexible, context-specific HIA approach to projects, programmes and policies has come about. This was raised by respondents in phase II of the study. The newly evolved HIA approach seems to be more fit for purpose. In the RoI a key change is the upcoming incorporation of HIA within SIA as outlined in the *Healthy Ireland* (2013) strategy. As noted already in this volume, if the focus is on the outcome (the outcome being improved considerations of health impacts for projects, programmes and policies) then how we arrive at that destination is of less relevance than arriving there at all. That is to say, perhaps the evolution of HIA is 'healthier' in terms of it being more suitable and pragmatic for use within policy development in the broadest sense.

This section presents the conclusions from across the four HIAs under study that are relevant to the practice of HIA in both jurisdictions.

The role of the health services and the meaning of health

Each of the HIAs under study reflected the importance of the meaning of health and the understanding of health inequalities and determinants of health. The social model of health is central to the HIA instrument and approach (Kemm and Parry, 2004). It was clear from this study that stakeholders in an HIA process must have a comprehension of such key underlying values of the policy-aiding mechanism, or at least a discussion could take place initially between stakeholders and partners regarding each individual's understanding of the key concepts.

HIA was considered a suitable instrument and approach to inform non-health service statutory stakeholders of the determinants of health, as identified by a respondent from Belfast Healthy Cities regarding the Belfast HIA.

It is an intersectoral instrument and approach capable of bringing various stakeholders together, as was illustrated in these four HIAs. This has also been highlighted in previous research by Davenport *et al.* (2006) as an intangible benefit of the HIA process. The lack of understanding of the social model of health concepts was deemed a barrier to the HIA process in the Donegal case, as pointed out by the Donegal Traveller Project. How institutions view health inequalities, and what value they place upon the concept, was deemed an important consideration in the Derry/Londonderry case. The reduction of health inequalities is the foundational rock of the HIA mechanism and its understanding is vital to the future development, understanding and success of the instrument and approach.

In the Ballyfermot HIA, numerous health promotion activities resulted from the HIA process, such as healthy eating campaigns at the local Tesco store, school health promotion programmes and the Cold Weather Response Initiative. This indicates a successful spillover effect, an incidental benefit that the process had for the local health services.

The drive to embed HIAs within the bureaucratic machinery of the HSE and PHA poses a challenge for the future, but it is necessary for the instrument and approach to become mainstreamed (Devlin, 2007; Wismar *et al.*, 2007), institutionalised (Banken, 2003) and used on a systematic basis if it is to develop as a credible and feasible policy-aiding tool (Kearns and Pursell, 2007). This drive and need for institutionalisation was highlighted by respondents from the former WIFH team in Northern Ireland, HSE in the Republic of Ireland and Institute of Public Health. A respondent from the Chartered Institute of Environmental Health Northern Ireland made the point that public health is much more than the health services, and if HIA is to be adequately mainstreamed and used, it needs to be mainstreamed across the sectors that have an interest in public health, such as local councils, environmental health officers, planning officials, transport and housing departments, and so on. Leadership could come from within the health services; however HIA will not be used to its maximum potential if it remains within the sole remit of the health services.

The support for the HIA instrument and approach within the health services is vital for its future development. All respondents from the health services who were involved in the HIA cases were fully supportive of the instrument and approach. However, an exploratory interview with a health promotion officer in the HSE Western Region of the Republic indicated how the dissatisfaction of one senior individual within the HSE can impact on the conduct of HIAs at an institutional level, as the senior individual was identified as a self-confessed critic of HIAs being conducted. Institutional leadership, high-level support, or non-support, plays an important role for the institutionalisation of HIAs within the health services. In order to ensure a greater level of objectivity for HIA and the process, and it not being dependent on enthusiastic champions, it needs to be mainstreamed through legislative mechanisms.

The role of actors in public policy

The involvement of key policy-makers and individuals informing policy development within the main institutional bodies that would use the HIA knowledge to formulate policy was integral to the process. However, the involvement of such individuals was not without difficulty or strain.

Partnership working between the various organisations and interests proved a frustrating battle in the Belfast HIA case, as although people came to the table in the end, there was a lack of willingness to share information and an entrenchment of institutional attitudes was endemic across the statutory stakeholders. The reform programme for local government may reduce these tensions, especially as local authorities gain more functions. The transfer of additional planning and regeneration functions will ensure the councils are the main decision-makers and this should ensure greater ease in conducting future HIAs.

The role of policy entrepreneurs (enthusiastic champions for HIA) was cited as an enabler in the cases; an individual within the local authority who had the motivation, vision and decision-making capacities to push the HIA agenda forward in their relevant institutional setting. Political and institutional leadership was deemed the determining factor in the success of the HIA by Belfast Healthy Cities respondents for the Belfast HIA. The meeting with innovative 'policy entrepreneurs' was cited as a bonus in this case study as well as in the Donegal, Dublin and Derry/Londonderry cases. Involving the appropriate individuals in the HIA, who are coming from an appropriate decision-making tier in their home institution with capacities to make and inform decisions, was vital to the success of the Derry/Londonderry case. The need for senior level commitment and statutory recognition were identified as key factors for the integration of policy-makers into the HIA process.

Engaging with the community in an HIA

> Then build people. Anyone can build buildings. (Browne in McSheffrey, 2000: 111)

Previous HIA research has cited the importance of community input and community development approaches to the HIA processes (Mittelmark *et al.*, 2007; Wismar *et al.*, 2007). The HIA instrument and approach was cited by respondents across the cases as enabling community mobilisation (Ballyfermot), fostering a bottom-up community development approach within the county council (Donegal), tapping into fragmented community infrastructure and facilitating its growth (Belfast), and enabling community consultation on issues that were never before brought to the residential community (Derry/Londonderry). highfalutin language and the use of technocratic jargon were cited as barriers for the full engagement of community representatives in the HIA at the beginning of the processes in both Ballyfermot and Derry/Londonderry, but both community respondents ensured that all stakeholders kept verbal communication at an appropriate level that was understandable to everyone. It was clear, despite the immovability of some statutory stakeholders in the Donegal case particularly, that 'communities shaping their own communities' and the empowerment that resulted from this ensured the sustainability of community involvement in the HIA issues when the official process had ended. This is evidenced in the Ballyfermot HIA where the LAG (known locally as the Impact Group) was restarted in September 2008 under the direction of the RAPID programme. Although it does not exist today, it influenced and informed a variety of local initiatives; in Donegal the Travelling community health researchers used their interviewing skills that were learned during the HIA for data collection of the Traveller national health survey; in Belfast local primary schools promoted clean air programmes and have tree-planting areas on site; and in Derry/Londonderry local residents had a role on the design and implementation team of the regeneration project. These are the often intangible benefits of an HIA that ensure sustainability of community involvement in local policy development.

Indeed as cited by a stakeholder in the Derry/Londonderry case, HIA is an appropriate instrument and approach to encourage partnership working across all stakeholders, which includes the community groups that will be affected by policy; the policy receivers. Cross-sectoral cooperation and mutual learning are important outcomes from the HIA processes in encouraging community empowerment and activity, as 'theoretical planning expertise is of little significance in the absence of community resolution' (McSheffrey, 2000: 109).

The question posed in Chapter 2 referred to whether the two 'faces of HIA could co-exist without negating one another' (O'Mullane, 2013: 30). These two 'faces' refer to the role HIA plays in generating scientific evidence, and in fostering community participation and enabling community knowledge and evidence to be presented within an HIA. It has been shown in the four HIAs that this is possible to a degree. However an important consideration are the expectations of stakeholders involved, which need to be clarified at the beginning of the process so as to avoid disappointment and tensions arising later in the process. In the four HIAs, it was shown that community participation led to sustainable outcomes, such as the Impact Group formation after the HIA was completed, and even after this group dissolved, a variety of initiatives were cited as being developed as a direct result of the HIA based on community identified needs.

The role of local government

As highlighted in Chapter 3, there are a variety of reforms and changes upcoming in the local government systems in both jurisdictions. The integration of HIA and similar health-proofing and policy-informing approaches with daily operations and within structural reform is very much in a state of flux. The lay of the land, as it were, will become much clearer once these changes are implemented. The amalgamation of local authorities in Northern Ireland (from twenty-six to eleven) and the reduction of the number of councillors (from 582 to 462) from April 2015 will bring about massive structural change, as well as the increase in the powers and functions of the authorities. In the Republic of Ireland, the amalgamation of some councils (Tipperary, Limerick and Waterford) and the abolition of town councils will reduce local authorities from 114 to 31, as legislated in the Local Government Reform Act 2014. Also the CDBs (where some health consultative functions lay and which mostly house the Healthy City projects) will be abolished and reformed under the Local Community Development Committees. Whether these changes will ensure greater cohesiveness of public health agendas at the local government level remains to be seen.

The tier of government that all the HIA cases operated in was at the local government level. This tier of government is most appropriate for the maximum use of HIA evidence for policy formulation (Elliott and Francis, 2005; Davenport *et al.*, 2006; Ison, 2007). The majority of HIAs conducted on the island of Ireland are carried out at this level. Therefore, the role that local government plays, as a state player in local decision-making, is an important consideration for the development of HIA into the future (O'Mullane and Quinlivan, 2012). Kearns and Pursell (2007) also concluded that the role of local government, in an Irish context, was an important one to understand in order for the use of HIAs in policy to be maximised. The Welsh policy document 'The route to health improvement: an organisational package to build capacity for local authorities' (2004) is a good example of how local authorities may work towards integrating health considerations into their intersectoral policy development, and HIA is a workable tool for such integration and sectoral collaboration.

The Belfast HIA case study illustrated that there is greater transparency and accountability at local government level which is lacking in the central government agencies in Northern Ireland. The lack of uniformity of policy agendas was a hindrance to the use of HIAs at local level in Northern Ireland. However many respondents noted the unequal role that exists between central and local government, during phase I of the study. In phase II of the study, it was clear that the reform proposed in the local government reform programme (which resulted from the RPA process) will introduce changes and measures to the benefit of local government, most notably (and importantly for HIA development), the transfer of planning and regeneration functions to local authorities from April 2015. It should be noted also that BCC is the largest and most resourced local authority in the jurisdiction and can access the support and input from Belfast Healthy Cities more easily than smaller, less resourced local authorities outside of the Belfast area can. This was raised in interviews in phase II. If HIA and the HiAP approach is hoped to be equally mainstreamed across all authorities, it needs to happen with an equal level of access to support, knowledge and expertise. Perhaps with the amalgamation of local authorities, the experience and expertise in HIA and associated approaches will be shared and pooled. Only time will tell if this will be the case.

The current political and administrative reform movement ongoing, within the framework of the RPA, has added a degree of uncertainty for the statutory stakeholders that are operating in the policy spheres. This was the case during phase I of the study and, again, it arose as a topic of discussion in phase II. To some extent HIA and its progress has been overshadowed by the reform agenda within the PHA, which, even though it was established in 2009, is still acclimatising to the structural and personnel changes, and at the time of writing, the public health framework is due but has not yet been released. In phase I of the study, respondents expressed uncertainty about the future implementation of the RPA, and in phase II, the PHA staff were still acclimatising to the changes and awaited the implementation of the reform of local government from April 2015. This uncertainty was evident in the Derry/Londonderry case, for example. However, Derry City Council played a ceremonial role at best in the HIA on Dove Gardens estate, whilst BCC was a key partner in the use and ownership of the HIA on the Draft Air Quality Action Plan.

Local government was identified as an appropriate setting for health considerations to be incorporated into local policy-making. The consultative and health dimension that HIA employed was deemed amenable for use at local authority level by those interviewed in the Northern Ireland HIAs.

The Donegal HIA highlighted the importance of political will in the local authority in advancing the path with a particular policy stance; in this case it was Traveller accommodation. The local mindset that was noted during the interview stage of the Donegal HIA was evidenced by local electoral politics, with the highly politicised launch of the HIA amongst local councillors, which then resulted in a lack of political cognisance or action taken with the findings of the HIA in the years after the HIA was completed. Then for the TAPs that commenced in 2009 and 2014, the HIA was included to some extent, though the practical implementation of the findings remains to be seen. The important role that Donegal County Council played in ensuring the HIA evidence was used or not was obvious. It was clear that the perception of the non-council respondents was that the council acted as a barrier in the full implementation of the Traveller Accommodation Policy, and in adopting new measures that would promote the health and wellbeing of accommodation centres. The subject topic of this HIA (Traveller accommodation) took over as the overriding factor in the experience of that HIA process.

In the Ballyfermot HIA, the central role that DCC played, and the importance of having council officials around the HIA, was of undeniable importance. Respondents in this process stated that the cross-sectoral cooperation and learning that came from the HIA process was beneficial to the conduct of local government business and amenable to the consultative policy environment, which is characteristic of present-day activities and values in consensual policy-making. URBAN II team members reiterated this point and stated that local government reform and the process of community consultation was facilitated by the workability of the HIA. This was also concluded in the research carried out under the auspices of the European HIA effectiveness research (Lavin and Metcalfe, 2007a).

The HIAs under study clearly indicate the importance of the role that local government plays, as an enabler in the HIA process (Belfast; Dublin), as a barrier (Donegal) and as an indifferent player in the process (Derry). In the Dublin and Belfast HIAs, the local authority played important dual roles as both owner and user of the HIA, whereas Donegal County Council was not an owner of the HIA (Donegal Traveller Project was leading the process but the majority of the recommendations were expected to be implemented by the council) but was the expected user. Derry City Council played a ceremonial role. The absence of such a vital partner was realised further down the HIA road at the design stage of the regeneration project. Since phase I of the study, Derry/Londonderry has since become a WHO designated Healthy City and this brings with it great potential for HIA to be mainstreamed and used more regularly. In research conducted by Davenport *et al.* (2006) the decision-makers having ownership of the HIA process was an enabler in the process, and this was clearly the case also in this study. The more ownership those making the policy decisions had over the HIA, the more likely the HIA would be used for policy.

The planning services: a vital partner

A significant finding from this study is the vital role the planning services play in the conduct and implementation of HIAs. It was clear from each HIA under study that the genuine involvement and commitment of planning officials to the HIA was a determining factor for the success in each case. This has been identified by HIA experts in the field (Barton, 2007; Birley and Birley, 2007). Planners are viewed as the 'gateway' to the processes of infrastructural and social development by HIA practitioners and academic experts (Cave, 2007). This point was highlighted in this study also.

Whilst in the RoI planning services are a function of local government, they were a separate entity in NI during the conduct of the HIAs on the Air Quality Action Plan and the regeneration of Dove Gardens estate. However from April 2015 this will change and local authorities will become the main decision-makers in planning. This transfer of functions (and more, including responsibilities regarding regeneration and some roads functions) could pave the way for smoother intersectoral work around developments and can enable great use of instruments such as HIA. The Community Planning aspect of the local government reform will be an interesting one, and one that HIA can definitely work within.

To legislate or not to legislate? The future for HIA

Recommendations were made throughout this study for the development of a type of IIA. This IIA instrument would amalgamate the main tenets of impact assessment frameworks that currently inhabit policy-making circles (environmental, health, social, equality, poverty, regulatory), as many are analogous and have the capacity for being joined-up (Lyons, 2005). This was suggested by respondents in the HIA cases, as well as by respondents from the health services and local government bodies, such as the PHA, HSE and Institute of Public Health. The respondent from the Chartered Institute of Environmental Health Northern Ireland succinctly summed it up by saying that if HIA is optional, then it stays optional.

HIA could be institutionalised via a type of IIA from a central government level initially, and mainstreamed at the local level secondly. To some extent this is happening, in that HIA will be incorporated within a SIA in the Republic, and is already included as part of the Policy Toolkit although it is currently only used at central government level NI. The degree to which HIA will be incorporated, and the way it will exist within SIA in the Republic remains to be seen.

The lack of mainstreaming has been identified as a barrier to the development of HIA in this book by respondents in all the HIAs under study, as in other research (Elliott and Francis, 2005; Davenport *et al.*, 2006). Discussions with planning officials throughout the study's research, in particular with senior planners, leads to the conclusion that for HIAs to become systematic and standardised throughout policy-making processes, and without adding to the workload of officials, an integration of health impacts and considerations may be the most pragmatic and realistic route. Some HIA purists fear this move (Scott-Samuel, 2006), as it may result in a dilution of the health focus. However, the integration of all impact assessment frameworks would ensure health impacts of policy are considered and it would be the most assessable route towards legislation of the tool.

Taking action: suggestions for the integration of HIA at local and national levels

The following includes practical suggestions for the development of HIA based on the lessons arising from the practice of the HIAs in this book's study.

Local level

There is capacity for the coordination of resources and strategic vision across the local government and health service institutions. Horizontal ways of working in partnership would enhance the workability of HIA, as well as increasing the role for evidence-based policy-making. Local authority and health service strategic planning has the potential to guarantee greater coordination of resources and to reduce duplication of work. The following are a number of recommendations for HIA development into the future, based on the findings of this book's study:

1. The local authority could be involved in the HIA from the beginning of process. This would maximise the use and ownership of the process and outcomes.
2. The health services have a key role to play in leading, coordinating and mainstreaming HIAs in both jurisdictions, and a responsibility to involve key stakeholders in the process.
3. Support for individuals initiating or seeking to initiate an HIA must be provided. This support could come from the Institute of Public Health, the government ministries and the implementation structures for the most recent public health frameworks in both jurisdictions.
4. Enable the initiation of networks which bring together professionals, on a voluntary basis, from sectors such as the health services, environmental health, academia and planning, who have an interest in conducting HIAs, such as the Southern HIA Network (network mostly for Cork city and county) in the RoI (Institute of Public Health in Ireland, 2010).
5. The Healthy City initiative is a workable and appropriate 'home' for embedding HIA as an instrument to promote health and wellbeing in the context of people's lives across both jurisdictions at the local level.

National level

Institutional leadership and political will have been identified in this book as necessary enablers for the feasibility and advancement of HIA. This was the conclusion in another similarly themed volume (O'Mullane, 2013). Such higher-level advocacy and support for the practice and use of HIAs into the future is required. This would ensure longevity for the policy-aiding instrument and approach. The implementation structures for the public health frameworks need to ensure this support, a necessary ingredient for HIA sustainability.

Conclusion

This book was written at an appropriate time juncture, essentially between the release and partial implementation of public health strategies in each jurisdiction and during a time when local government reform was conceptualised and partially implemented. Only time can reveal the impact of such structural changes on the conduct of HIA and its use for policy development. However if the most recent changes encourage greater cohesion in how HIAs are conducted, nurture the training and experiential learning around the practice of HIA and associated approaches, improve intersectoral working and learning, then they will only improve the development of healthier public policies for the island's populations. This book sought to present a picture of HIA in both jurisdictions along with generalisable lessons learned from the development of HIA as a policy support instrument and approach based on empirical data.

When combining the theoretical and empirical findings of this book's study, the overall conclusion is that HIAs are used in policy development. Now what is required is action whilst taking cognisance of the influences on HIA evidence use and the degrees to which the evidence can be used. For the implementation of the measures for HIA, the triadic approach to nurturing HIA throughout both jurisdictions as suggested by Gillespie and McIldoon (2009) would prove a good strategy, as demonstrated also by the findings in this book. First, HIA needs to be mainstreamed in all public health activities (which includes the actions affecting public health within local authorities); second, capacity-building in HIA must continue; and third, political will and leadership from the highest levels are required in order to ensure the support for the implementation of HIA.

Practically speaking, HIA use is influenced by the tier of government (local), the involvement of key partners and intersectoral action around the promotion of health and wellbeing, the conceptualisation of health, the role of the policy-makers and the community who will be on the receiving end of the policy/programme/project proposal. The development of a more pragmatic and tailored HIA approach being conducted in Northern Ireland provides an interesting example of how the instrument is evolving in an organic manner, and provides an example of how HIA can proceed into the future. In order to maximise the HIA process, a multidisciplinary network of representatives from statutory, voluntary, community bodies, and research institutions, with an interest in HIA should be formed. Such networks can be coordinated, although not exclusively, by the health services. A partnership approach to working is required for the maximum advancement of the HIA concept.

It is clear that the extent of such use varies, and a linear and rational investigation of HIA use in policy development that focused on direct instrumental utilisation alone would have proven superficial and lacking depth. This is why an examination of the indirect (conceptual and persuasive) use of HIAs was required. Certainly, this book has shown how 'HIA fits best within the often non-linear public policy cycle as a policy formulation instrument' (Harris *et al.*, 2014: 1). By examining the influences on the use of HIA evidence and knowledge, and investigating the relationship between the influences, the extent of the use and the congruence of these theories and schools of literature with the findings, all cases displayed conceptual use of HIA for policy formulation. This indicates the conclusion that the instrument and approach does impact on policy development and can be used instrumentally in the future. The Ballyfermot, Belfast and Derry/Londonderry cases indicated instrumental use of the HIA. During phase I of the study, instrumental use in the Donegal case was not found. However, during phase II the HIA was found to have been used instrumentally within the subsequent programmes; however the jury is still out on the concrete implementation of the HIA recommendations. This is a limitation of the study and framework, not being in a position to establish the exact instrument use, and only a full-scale evaluation of that HIA would establish the number of recommendations that were implemented. The difficulties in establishing the use of the HIA for policy development may be more related to the topic of Traveller accommodation being implicitly controversial than the infeasibility of the HIA instrument. The Donegal, Belfast and Derry/Londonderry HIAs under study indicated their use was of a persuasive nature. This would concur with previous research, whereby the HIA can lead to 'a politicisation of knowledge rather than to the rationalisation of policy' (Bekker, 2007: 194). The study in this book has provided greater insight to the influences on HIA utilisation in policy, and more specifically, the extent of that utilisation. This volume indicates that the use of HIAs is influenced by its contextual conditions which could be foreseen prior to project commencement and would therefore enable a smoother and enlightened process.

Harris *et al.* (2014: 1) make a good point and are backed up by the findings and conclusions of this book:

> HIAs for policy are necessarily both tactical and technical. Within policy subsystems using HIA to influence public policy requires tactically positioning health as a relevant public policy issue and, to facilitate this, institutional support for collaboration between Public Health and other sectors. HIA provides,

tactically and technically, a space for practical reasoning to navigate facts, values and processes underlying the substantive and procedural dimensions of policy.

The HIAs in this book were conducted in order to influence policy development in some shape or form. The HIAs provided a space for negotiation, intersectoral communication and collaborations, and ensured one more gateway to the policy process by tactically placing health on the policy agenda and, technically, in generating an evidence base to be used within policy development. This concept of HIA provides a useful way of viewing HIA in its future advancement.

For the advancement and flourishing of the instrument and approach, it must be recognised that no process partner may work alone on an HIA. What is required is a partnership approach to working with a pooling of resources, expertise, experience and interest, and a respectful understanding of varying perspectives and views. Without the high-level political and institutional support for HIA, the instrument and the evidence it provides will be destined for dusty shelves. The time for HIA has come. It is up to those involved in the advancement and nurturing of the process to stand up to the challenge of furthering better informed and inclusive policy-making.

Bibliography

Acheson, D. (1998) *Inequalities in Health: Report of an Independent Inquiry*, London: HMSO.

Adelle, C. and Weiland, S. (2012) 'Policy assessment and the state of the art', *Impact Assessment and Project Appraisal*, 30 (1), pp. 25–33.

Atkinson, P. and Cooke, A. (2005) 'Developing a framework to assess the costs and benefits of health impact assessment', *Environmental Impact Assessment Review*, 25, pp. 791–8.

Bachrach, P.S. and Baratz, M.S. (1970) *Power and Poverty: Theory and Practice*, New York: Oxford University Press.

Bacigalupe, A., Esnaola, S., Calderón, C., Zuazagoitia, J. and Aldasoro, E. (2010) 'Health impact assessment of an urban regeneration project: opportunities and challenges in the context of a southern European city', *J Epidemiol Community Health*, 64, pp. 950–5.

Bambra, C., Fox, D. and Scott-Samuel, A. (2007) 'Towards a politics of health', in Douglas, J., Earle, S., Handsley, S., Lloyd, C. and Spurr, S. (eds) *A Reader in Promoting Public Health: Challenge and Controversy*, London: Sage and Open University.

Banken, R. (2001) *Strategies for Institutionalising HIA*, Brussels: European Centre for Health Policy.

Banken, R. (2003) 'Health Impact Assessment: how to start the process and make it last', *Bulletin of the World Health Organisation*, 81 (3), p. 389.

Barrington, R. (1987) *Health, Medicine and Politics in Ireland 1900–1970*, Dublin: Irish Public Administration.

Barton, H. (2007) 'A settlement health map', *Town and Country Planning-Special Issue*, 76 (2), pp. 47–9.

Barton, H. and Grant, M. (2006) 'A health map for the local human habitat', *The Journal for the Royal Society for the Promotion of Health*, 126 (6), pp. 252–3.

Barton, H. and Tsourou, C. (2000) *Healthy Urban Planning*, London and New York: Spon Press on behalf of the World Health Organization.

Baum, F., Ollila, E. and Pena, S. (2013) 'History of health in all policies', in Leppo, K., Ollila, E., Pena, S., Wismar, M. and Cook, S. (eds) *Health in All Policies, Seizing Opportunities, Implementing Policies*, Finland: Ministry of Social Affairs and Health, Department for Promotion of Welfare and Health.

Bekker, M. (2007) *The Politics of Healthy Policies: Redesigning HIA to Integrate Health in Public Policy*, Postbus, The Netherlands: Eburon Delft.

Bekker, M.P.M., Putters, K. and Van der Grinten, T.E.D. (2004) 'Exploring the relations between evidence and decision-making: a political-administrative approach to health impact assessment', *Environmental Impact Assessment Review*, 24, pp. 139–49.

Bekker, M.P.M., Putters, K. and Van der Grinten, E.D. (2005) 'Evaluating the impact of Health Impact Assessment on urban reconstruction decision-making: who manages whose risks?', *Environmental Impact Assessment Review*, 25 (7–8), pp. 758–71.

Belfast City Council (2006) *Belfast City Air Quality Action Plan*, Belfast: Pollutant Control Section, Belfast City Council.

Belfast Healthy Cities (2007a) *Health Impacts of Regeneration: Issue 1*, Planning for Healthier People, September, Belfast: BHC.

Belfast Healthy Cities (2007b) *Health Impact Assessment; Healthy Urban Planning, Belfast Healthy Cities*, information folder on the work of the organisation, Belfast: BHC.

Bhatia, R. and Corburn, J. (2011) 'Lessons from San Francisco: health impact assessments have advanced political conditions for improving population health', *Health Affairs*, 30 (12), pp. 2410–18.

Birley, M. (2003) 'Health impact assessment: integration and critical appraisal', *Impact Assessment and Project Appraisal*, 21 (4), pp. 313–21.

Birley, M. (2011) *Health Impact Assessment: Principles and Practice*, London: Earthscan.

Birley, M. and Birley, V. (2007) *Healthy Design Principles for Use in the HIA of Mixed Residential Developments*, Birley HIA, Health Impact Association.

Birrell, D. and Hayes, A. (1999) *The Local Government System in Northern Ireland*, Dublin: Irish Public Administration.

Blakely, T., Baker, M.G. and Howden-Chapman, P. (2011) 'Commentary: does housing policy influence health?', *J Epidemiol Community Health*, 65, pp. 598–9.

Boldo, E., Linares, C., Lumbreras, J., Borge, R., Narros, A., Garcia-Perez, J., Fernandez-Navarro, P., Perez-Gomez, B., Aragones, N., Ramis, R., Pollan, M., Moreno, T., Karanasiou, A. and Lopez-Abente G. (2011) 'Health impact assessment of a reduction in ambient PM2.5 levels in Spain', *Environment International*, 37 (2), pp. 342–8.

Bond, A., Morrison-Saunders, A. and Pope, J. (2012) 'Sustainability assessment: the state of the art', *Impact Assessment and Project Appraisal*, 30 (1), pp. 53–62.

Bond, A., Cave, B. and Ballantyne, R. (2013) 'Who plans for health improvement? SEA, HIA and the separation of spatial planning and health planning', *Environmental Impact Assessment Review*, 42, pp. 67–73.

Bonner, B. (2007) 'HIA Dove Gardens: a personal experience', *HIA Forum, Institute of Public Health*, April, Newry, Co. Down, Northern Ireland.

Bonner, B. (2011) *HIA – Dove Gardens: Turning Theory into Practice*, Public Health Agency, Northern Ireland. Version 4.0.

Bos, R. (2006) 'Health impact assessment and health promotion', *Bull World Health Organ*, 84, pp. 914–15.

Cahill, D. (2012) *Health Promotion in Ireland – Examples from Practice*, Guest lecture presentation given to Trnava University public health doctoral candidates, 2 February 2012 (web presentation).

Carley, M.J. (1980) *Rational Techniques in Policy Analysis*, London: Heinemann Educational Books.

Cashmore, M. Richardson, T., Hilding-Ryedvik, T. and Emmelin, L. (2010) 'Evaluating the effectiveness of impact assessment instruments: theorising the nature and implications of their political constitution', *Environmental Impact Assessment Review*, 30, pp. 371–9.

Cave, B. (2007) 'Building in health: assessing the potential effects on health of a strategic urban extension in Devon', 8th International HIA Conference, *Healthy Public Policy – Is HIA the Cornerstone?* Dublin Castle, Ireland, 16–17 October.

Cave, B., Jha-Thakur, U., Rao, M., Labhasetwar, P. and Fischer, T. (2013) 'Health in impact assessment and emerging challenges in India', in O'Mullane, M. (ed.) *Integrating Health Impact Assessment with the Policy Process: Lessons and Experiences from around the World*, Oxford: Oxford University Press.

CAWT (2014) Personal correspondence with a member of the organisation, 5 March 2014.

Central Statistics Office (CSO) (2013) 'Population, 1901–2011', available at: www.cso.ie/Quicktables/GetQuickTables.aspx?FileName=CNA13.asp&TableName=Population+1901+-+2011&StatisticalProduct=DB_CN, accessed 13 February 2014.

Chelimsky, E. (1995) 'Where we stand today in the practice of evaluation: some reflections', *Knowledge and Policy*, 8 (3), pp. 8–20.

Clancy, I., Goodman, P., Sinclair, H. and Dockery, D.W. (2002) 'Effect of air pollution control on death rates in Dublin, Ireland: an intervention study', *Lancet*, 360, pp. 1210–14.

Clarke, J., Langan, M. and Williams, F. (2001) 'The construction of the British welfare state, 1945–1975', in Cochrane, A., Clarke, J. and Gewirtz, S. (eds) *Comparing Welfare States*, 2nd edn, London, Newbury and New Delhi: Sage.

Commission on Social Determinants of Health (2008) *CSDH Final Report: Closing the Gap in a Generation: Health Equity through Action on the Social Determinants of Health*, Geneva: World Health Organization.

Community Workers Cooperative (2006) *Bulletin of the CWC*, Issue No. 2, July, Tuam Road, Galway: CWC News.

Community Workers Cooperative (2007) *Donegal Community Workers Cooperative*, available at: www.cwc.ie/about/donegal.html.

Cooper, R., Boyko, C. and Codinhoto, R. (2009) 'The effect of the physical environment on mental wellbeing', in Cooper, C.L., Field, J., Goswami, U., Jenkins, R. and Sahakian, B.J. (eds) *Mental Capital and Wellbeing*, New Jersey: Wiley-Blackwell.

Corvalan, C., Briggs, D. and Zielhuis, G. (eds) (2000) *Decision Making in Environmental Health: From Evidence to Action*, Geneva: WHO.

Cross, M., Henke, R., Oberknezev, P. and Pouliasi, K. (2000) *Towards Effective Means of Linking Scientific Research and Public Policy: Migrants in European Cities*, Utrecht: Netherlands School for Social and Economic Research.

Council of the European Union (2006) 'Council conclusions on health in all policies (HiAP)', 2767th Employment, Social Policy, Health and Consumer Affairs Council Meeting, Brussels.

Daeman, H. and Schaap, L. (2000) 'Ireland: associated democracy', In Daeman, H.F.M. and Schaap, L. (eds) *Citizen and City: Developments in Fifteen Local Democracies in Europe*, Rotterdam: Centre for Local Democracy.

Dahlgren, G. and Whitehead, M. (1991) *Policies and Strategies to Promote Social Equity in Health*, Stockholm: Institute for Future Studies.

Davenport, C., Mathers, J. and Parry, J. (2006) 'Use of health impact assessment in incorporating health considerations in decision making', *Journal of Epidemiology and Community Health*, 60, pp. 196–201.

Davies, C. (2000) 'Understanding the policy process', in Brechin, A., Brown, H. and Eby, M.A. (eds) *Critical Practice and Social Care*, London: Sage.

Deelstra, Y., Nooteboom, S.G., Kohlmann, H.R., van den Berg, J. and Innanen, S. (2003) 'Using knowledge for decision making purposes in the context of large projects in the Netherlands', *Environmental Impact Assessment Review*, 23, pp. 517–41.

De Nazelle, A., Rodriguez, D.A. and Crawford-Brown, D. (2009) 'The built environment and health: impacts of pedestrian-friendly designs on air pollution exposure', *Science of the Total Environment*, 407 (8), pp. 2525–35.

Department of the Environment (1996) *Better Local Government: A Programme for Change*, Dublin: The Stationery Office.

Department of the Environment (2013a) *Local Government Reform*, Belfast: Department of the Environment Northern Ireland, available at: www.doeni.gov.uk/benefits_of_local_government_reform.pdf, accessed 17 February 2014.

Department of the Environment (2013b) *Local Government Reform Guidance to Councils: Community Planning Foundation Programme*, Belfast: Department of the Environment Local Government Policy Division.

Department of the Environment, Community and Local Government (2013) *Local Government Reform: Putting People First: Action Programme for Effective Local Government*, available at: www.environ.ie/en/LocalGovernment/LocalGovernmentReform/, accessed 11 February 2014.

Department of Health (2010) All-Ireland Traveller Health Study, Dublin: Stationery Office, available at: www.dohc.ie/publications/traveller_health_study.html, accessed 10 December 2013.

Department of Health (2012) *Health in Ireland, Key Trends 2012*, Dublin: Department of Health, Information Unit.

Department of Health (2013) *Healthy Ireland: Framework for Improved Health and Well-being, 2013 to 2025*, Dublin: Department of Health.

Department of Health and Children (2001) *Quality and Fairness: A Health System for You*, Dublin: The Stationery Office.

Department of Health Social Services and Public Safety (DHSSPS) (2002) *Investing for Health*, Belfast: Department of Health, Social Services and Public Safety.

Department of Health Social Services and Public Safety (DHSSPS) (2005) *A Healthier Future: A Twenty Year Vision for Health and Wellbeing in Northern Ireland, 2005–2025*, Belfast: Department of Health, Social Services and Public Safety.

Department of Health Social Services and Public Safety (DHSSPS) (2013) *Consultation on 'Fit and Well – Changing Lives – A Ten Year Public Health Strategic Framework for Northern Ireland 2012–2022'*, available at: www.dhsspsni.gov.uk/showconsultations?txtid=57771, accessed 17 February 2014.

Department of Health Social Services and Public Safety (DHSSPS) (2014) *Making Life Better – A Whole System Framework for Public Health 2013–2023*, available at: www.dhsspsni.gov.uk/making-life-better.htm, accessed 12 July 2014.

Department of Social and Family Affairs (2006) *Report on Consultation for National Action Plan against Poverty and Social Exclusion 2006–2008*, Office for Social Inclusion. Dublin: The Stationery Office, available at: www.socialinclusion.ie/Report_Consultation_2006-2008.html, accessed 2 March 2014.

Derry City Council (2014) *Statutory Transition Committee appoint John Kelpie to the post of the Chief Executive Designate for the new Derry City and Strabane District Council*, available at: www.derrycity.gov.uk/News/Statutory-Transition-Committee-appoint-John-Kelpie, accessed 3 March 2014.

Devlin, J. (2007) 'Mainstreaming HIA in the WHO Healthy Cities Network', 8th Health Impact Assessment Conference, Dublin Castle Ireland, 17 October.

Devlin, J. (2013) 'Healthy cities: innovation, leadership and shared governance', paper presented at the First EcCoWell Conference, Cork, Ireland, 26 September 2013. Available at: http://eccowellcork.com/wp-content/uploads/2013/10/Joan-Devlin.pdf, accessed 19 January 2014.

Doherty, T. (2006) 'The way forward', in Lindsay, S. (ed.) *Health in Our Hands, A Celebration of Achievement: Summary of Ex-Post Evaluation 2001 to 2006 of the Bogside and Brandywell Health Forum*, Derry: Bogside and Brandywell Health Forum.

Donegal County Council (2004) *Housing Services Donegal County Council*, available at: www.donegalcoco.ie/services/housing/, accessed 12 March 2014.

Donegal Local Development Company (DLDC) (2007) *Donegal Local Development Company*, available at: www.dldc.org/.

Donegal Travellers Project (2006) *Health Impact Assessment of the Accommodation Programme for Travellers 2005–2008 for Donegal*, Donegal: DTP.

Dora, C. (2004) 'HIA in strategic environmental assessment and its application to policy in Europe', in Kemm, J., Parry, J. and Palmer, S. (eds) *Health Impact Assessment: Concepts, Theories, Techniques and Applications*, Oxford: Oxford University Press.

Douglas, M. and Scott-Samuel, A. (2001) 'Addressing health inequalities in health impact assessment', *Journal of Epidemiology and Community Health*, 55, pp. 450–1.

Douglas, M., Palmer, S. and Higgins, M. (2013) 'Integrating health into impact assessments in Scotland', in O'Mullane, M. (ed.) *Integrating Health Impact Assessment with the Policy Process: Lessons and Experiences from around the World*, Oxford: Oxford University Press.

Douglas, M., Thompson, H., Jepson, R., Hurley, M., Muirie, J. and Gorman, D. (2007) *Health Impact Assessment of Transport Initiatives: A Guide*, Edinburgh: NHS Health Scotland.

Doyle, C. (2006) 'Health Impact Assessment of Travellers' Accommodation Programme 2005–2008 in Donegal', *7th International Health Impact Assessment Conference*, Cardiff, Wales, 5–6 April.

Dublin City Council (2001) *URBAN II Ireland: Community Initiative Programme, 2000–2006*, Dublin: Dublin City Council.

Dublin City Council (2004) *Ballyfermot Air Quality and Noise Assessment*, Dublin: Traffic Noise and Air Quality Unit, Roads and Traffic Department, Dublin City Council.

Dye, T.R. (1976) *What Governments Do, Why They Do It, What Difference It Makes*, Alabama: Alabama University Press.

Eastern Regional Health Authority (ERHA) (2004) *A Health Impact Assessment of Traffic and Transport in Ballyfermot*, Dublin: ERHA.

EcCoWell Cork (2013) 'EcCoWell', *International EcCoWell Conference*, 26–27 September, Cork City.

Elliott, E. and Francis, S. (2005) 'Making effective links to decision-making: key challenges for Health Impact Assessment', *Environmental Impact Assessment Review*, 25 (7–8), pp. 747–57.

Elliott, E. and Williams, G. (2008) 'Developing public sociology through health impact assessment', *Sociology of Health & Illness*, 30 (7).

Engel, G.L. (1977) 'The need for a new medical model: a challenge for biomedicine', *Science*, 32, pp. 129–136.

Environmental Protection Agency (2002) *Guidelines on the Information to be Contained in the Environmental Impact Statement*, Wexford: EPA.

Eriksson, M. and Lindström, B. (2008) 'A salutogenic interpretation of the Ottawa Charter', *Health Promot Int.*, 23, pp. 190–9.

Esteves, A.M., Franks, D. and Vanclay, F. (2012) 'Social impact assessment: the state of the art', *Impact Assessment and Project Appraisal*, 30 (10), pp. 34–42.

European Centre of Public Health (ECPH) (1999) *Health Impact Assessment: Main Concepts and Suggested Approach, Gothenberg Consensus Paper*, Copenhagen: WHO Regional Office for Europe.

European Commission, The European Environment & Health Action Plan 2004–2010 COM (2004) Official Journal C 49.

Fabrizio, B. and Paolo, L. (2011) 'Health impact assessment: a multidisciplinary procedure to support decision making in public health', *Epidemiolgoia and Prevenzione*, 35 (2), pp. 73–6.

Fehr, R., Viliani, F., Nowacki, J. and Martuzzi, M. (2014) *Health in Impact Assessments: Opportunities not to be Missed*, Copenhagen: WHO Regional Office for Europe.

Fenwick, E., Macdonald, C. and Thomson, H. (2013) 'Economic analysis of the health impacts of housing improvement studies: a systematic review'. JECH Online First, published on 8 August 2013 as 10.1136.

FGS McClure Watters Consulting (2010) *Investing for Health Strategy Review, Final Report*. Prepared for the DHSSPS, Northern Ireland, available at: www.dhsspsni.gov.uk/health_development-final_report_-_september_2010.pdf, accessed 20 February 2014.

Frumkin, H., Frank, L. and Jackson, R. (2004) *Urban Sprawl and Public Health: Designing, Planning and Building for Healthy Communities*, Washington, DC: Island Press.

Fuller, L. (2004) *Irish Catholicism since 1950: The Undoing of a Culture*, Dublin: Gill and Macmillan.

Gagnon, F., Turgeon, J. and Dallaire, C. (2007) 'Healthy public policy: a conceptual cognitive framework', *Health Policy*, 81 (1), pp. 42–55.

Geelen, Loes M.J., Huijbregts, Mark A.J., Jans, Henk W.A., Ragas, A.M.J., Den Hollander, H.A. and Aben, J.M.M. (2013) 'Comparing the impact of fine particulate matter emissions from industrial facilities and transport on the real age of a local community', *Atmospheric Environment*, 73, pp. 138–44.

George, A.L. and Bennett, A. (2004) *Case Studies and Theory Development in the Social Sciences*, Cambridge, Massachusetts and London, England: MIT Press.

Gillespie, N. and McIldoon, N. (2009) *Final Report: Review of Health Impact Assessment for the Institute of Public Health in Ireland*, available at: www.publichealth.ie/sites/default/files/documents/files/Review%20of%20Health%20Impact%20Assessment%20in%20Ireland%202009.pdf, accessed 19 February 2014.

Glackin, D. and Farrell, B. (2006) *Health Impact Assessment Dove Gardens (Report)*, Derry: CAWT Development Centre.

Glackin, D., Farrell, B., Mason, C., Lavery, A., Burke, C. and Adams, B. (2006) 'An HIA of Northern Ireland Housing Executive proposal to redevelop Dove Gardens estate', *International HIA Conference*, Cardiff, Wales, 5 April.

Gorman, D., Douglas, M.J., Conway, L., Noble, P. and Hanlon, P. (2003) 'Transport policy and health inequalities: a health impact assessment of Edinburgh's transport policy', *Public Health*, 117, pp. 15–24.

Grow, H.M., Saelens, B.E., Kerr, J., Durant, N.H., Norman, G.J. and Sallis, J.F. (2008) 'Where are youth active? Roles of proximity, active transport, and built environment', *Medicine and Science in Sports and Exercise*, 40, pp. 2071–9.

Guba, E.G. and Lincoln, Y.S. (1989) *Fourth Generation Evaluation*, Newbury Park: Sage Publications.

Guliš, G. and Kollárová, J. (2013) 'Health impact assessment implementation and public health policy systems in Denmark and Slovakia', in O'Mullane, M. (ed.) *Integrating Health Impact Assessment with the Policy Process: Lessons and Experiences from around the World*, Oxford: Oxford University Press.

Guliš, G., Mekel, O., Ádám, B. and Cori, L. (2014) *Assessment of Population Health Risks of Policies*, New York: Springer.

Haggerty, B. and Melnick, A. (2013) 'Translating research to policy through health impact assessment in Clark County, Washington: a commentary to accompany the active living research', *Annals of Behavioural Medicine*, 25 (supplement 1), pp. S6–S8.

Hague, R. and Harrop, M. (2001) *Comparative Government and Politics*, 5th edn, Basingstoke: Palgrave Macmillan.

Ham, C. and Hill, M. (1993) *The Policy Process in the Modern Capitalist State*, London and New York: Harvester Wheatsheaf.

Harris, E. and Harris-Roxas, B. (2010) 'Health in all policies: a pathway for thinking about our broader societal goals', *Public Health Bull SA*, 7, pp. 43–6.

Harris, P. (2006) 'The driving forces for health impact assessment', *7th International Health Impact Assessment Conference*, Cardiff, Wales, 5–6 April.

Harris, P.J., Kemp, L.A. and Sainsbury, P. (2012) 'The essential elements of health impact assessment and healthy public policy: a qualitative study of practitioner perspectives', *BMJ Open*, 2, pp. 1–8.

Harris, P., Sainsbury, P. and Kemp, L. (2014) 'The fit between health impact assessment and public policy: practice meets theory', *Social Science & Medicine*, 108, pp. 46–53.

Harris-Roxas, B. and Harris, E. (2011) 'Differing forms, differing purposes: a typology of health impact assessment', *Environmental Impact Assessment Review*, 31 (4), pp. 396–403.

Harris-Roxas, B. and Harris, E. (2013) 'The impact and effectiveness of health impact assessment: a conceptual framework', *Environmental Impact Assessment Review*, 42, pp. 51–9.

Harris-Roxas, B., Viliani, F., Harris, P., Bond, A., Cave, B., Divall, M., Furu, P., Soeberg, M., Wernham, A. and Winkler, M. (2012) 'Health impact assessment: the state of the art', *Impact Assessment and Project Appraisal*, pp. 1–11.

Hayes, C. (2003) *Project Proposal Form: Health Impact Assessment of Traffic and Transport in Ballyfermot*, Dublin: ERHA (unpublished).

Hayes, C. (2006) 'Reflections on engaging with the HIA process: progressing HIA within the HSE', paper presentation. Institute of Public Health: Comprehensive Health Impact Assessment Training Course, 25–27 September, Malahide Court Hotel, Dublin.

Health Service Executive (HSE) (2006) *An Introduction to the HSE*, Dr. Steevens' Hospital, Dublin: Health Service Executive.

Health Services Executive (HSE) (2011) *Health Promotion Strategic Framework*, Dublin: HSE National Health Promotion Office.

Heclo, H. (1972) 'Review article: policy analysis', *British Journal of Political Science*, 2, pp. 83–108.

Hertwich, E.G. and Hammitt, J.K. (2000) 'A decision-analytic framework for impact assessment', *International Journal of Life-Cycle Assessment*, 5, pp. 5–12.

Hogwood, B.W. and Gunn, L.A. (1984) *Policy Analysis for the Real World*, Oxford: Oxford University Press.

Hood, C. (2002) 'The risk game and the blame game', *Government and Opposition*, 37 (1), pp. 15–54.

Howlett, M. and Ramesh, M. (2003) *Studying Public Policy: Policy Cycles and Policy Sub-Systems*, 2nd edn, Canada: Oxford University Press.

Howlett, M., Ramesh, M. and Perl, A. (2009) *Studying Public Policy: Policy Cycles and Policy Subsystems*, Oxford: Oxford University Press.

Hunt, P. (2007) 'Embedding HIA: sustainable approaches', 8th International HIA Conference, *Healthy Public Policy: Is HIA the Cornerstone?* Dublin Castle, Ireland, 16 October.

Immergut, E.M. (1992) 'The rule of the game: the logic of health policy making in France, Switzerland, and Sweden', in Steinmo, S., Thelen, K. and Longstreth, F. (eds) *Structuring Politics: Historical Institutionalism in Comparative Analysis*, Cambridge: Cambridge University Press.

Indecon International Consultants (2005) *Indecon Review of Local Government Financing*, Dublin: Indecon International Economic Consultants.

Institute of Public Health (2007) *Completed HIAs: Belfast City Air Quality Action Plan HIA*, Dublin and Belfast: Institute of Public Health Ireland, available at: www.publichealth.ie/index.asp?locID=127&docID=646.

Institute of Public Health in Ireland (2010) *Southern HIA Network*, available at: www.publichealth.ie/ireland/southernhia, accessed 11 March 2014.

Institute of Public Health in Ireland (2011) *About the Institute of Public Health in Ireland*, available at: www.publichealth.ie/about, accessed 18 February 2014.

Institute of Public Health in Ireland (2012) *New 10 Year Northern Ireland Public Health Framework – Consultation Launched*, available at: www.publichealth.ie/press-release/new-10-year-northern-ireland-public-health-framework-consultation-launched, accessed 18 February 2014.

Institute of Public Health in Ireland (2013) *Growing Health: Findings from a HIA on the North West Community Allotment/Garden Proposal*, Belfast: IPH.

International Association for Impact Assessment (2006) *Up, Down and Sideways: Extending and Integrating Assessments*, Irish-UK branch launch event, 24 March. University College Dublin.

Ison, E. (2006) *Health Impact Assessment of the Draft Air Quality Action Plan for Belfast*, (abridged version), Belfast: Belfast City Council (May).

Ison, E. (2009) 'The introduction of health impact assessment in the WHO European Healthy Cities Network', *Health Promotion International*, 24, pp. 64–71.

Ison, I. (2007) 'How to maximise HIA's influence on decision making and policy making at local government level', *Health Impact Assessment Seminar*, Galway Bay Hotel, Galway, Health Services Executive, West; National University of Ireland, Galway; Healthy Cities, Galway, 1 June 2007.

Jackson, R., Bear, D., Bhatia, R., Cantor, S.B., Cave, B., Diez Roux, A.V., Dora, C., Fielding, J.E., Zivin, J.S.G., Levy, J.I., Quint, J.I., Raja, S., Schulz, A.J. and Wernham, A.A. (2011) *Improving Health in the United States: The Role of Health Impact Assessment*, Washington DC: Committee on Health Impact Assessment. Board on Environmental Studies and Toxicology, Division on Earth and Life Studies, National Research Council of the National Academies. 2011. Available at: www.nap.edu/catalog.php?record_id=13229, accessed 21 February 2014.

Janowitz, M. (1970) 'Sociological models and social policy', in Janowitz, M., *Political Conflict: Essays in Political Sociology*, Chicago: Quadrangle Books.

Joffe, M. (2008) 'The need for strategic health assessment', *European Journal of Public Health*, 18 (5), pp. 436–40.

John, P. (1993) *Local Government in Northern Ireland*, York: Joseph Rowntree Foundation.

Jordan, A., McCall, J., Moore, W., Reid, H. and Stewart, D. (2006) *Health Systems in Transition: Northern Ireland*, Copenhagen: WHO Regional Office for Europe on behalf of the European Observatory on Health Systems and Policies.

Kavanagh, P., Doyle, C. and Metcalfe, O. (2005) *Health Impacts of Transport*, Dublin and Belfast: Institute of Public Health Ireland.

Kearns, N. and Pursell, L. (2007) *Evaluation of the HIA of Traffic and Transport in Ballyfermot*, Department of Health Promotion: National University of Ireland Galway.

Kearns, N. and Pursell, L. (2011) 'Time for a paradigm change? Tracing the institutionalisation of health impact assessment in the Republic of Ireland across health and environmental sectors', *Health Policy*, 99 (2), pp. 91–6.

Kelleher, C. (1999) 'Health and the Celtic Tiger: progress of health promotion in modern Ireland', *Health Education Research*, 14, pp. 151–4.

Kelly, I. and Clancy, L. (1984) 'Mortality in a general hospital and urban air pollution', *Irish Medical Journal*, 77 (10), pp. 322–4.

Kemm, J. (2001) 'Health Impact Assessment: a tool for healthy public policy', *Health Promotion International*, 16 (1).

Kemm, J. (2005) 'The future challenges for HIA', *Environmental Impact Assessment Review*, 25, pp. 799–807.

Kemm, J. (2006) 'Past and future of health impact assessment', *Comprehensive Health Impact Assessment Training Course*, Institute of Public Health, Malahide, Dublin, 25–27 September.

Kemm, J. (2011) 'HIA-advocacy or impartiality', 11th HIA International Conference, Granada, Spain, 14–15 April.

Kemm, J. (ed.) (2012) *Health Impact Assessment: Past Achievement, Current Understanding and Future Progress*, Oxford: Oxford University Press.

Kemm, J. and Parry, J. (2004) 'The development of health impact assessment', in Kemm, J., Parry, J. and Palmer, S. (eds) *Health Impact Assessment: Concepts, Theories, Techniques and Applications*, Oxford: Oxford University Press.

Kemm, J., den Broeder, L., Wismar, M., Fehr, R., Douglas, M. and Guliš, G. (2011) *How Can HIA Support Health in All Policies?* Draft document presented at the Poznan Meeting of the Polish Presidency, 8 November 2011.

Kickbusch, I., McCann, W. and Sherbon, T. (2008) 'Adelaide revisited: from healthy public policy to Health in All Policies', *Health Promotion International*, 23, pp. 1–4.

Knoepfel, P., Larrue, C., Varone, F. and Hill, M. (2007) *Public Policy Analysis*, Bristol: Policy Press.

Knox, C. (2003) 'Northern Ireland local government', in M. Callanan and J.F. Keogan (eds) *Local Government in Ireland: Inside Out*, Dublin: Institute of Public Administration.

Knox, C. (2008) 'Policy-making in Northern Ireland', *Policy and Politics*, 36 (3), pp. 343–59.

Knox, C. and Carmichael, P. (2005) 'Improving public services: public administration reform in Northern Ireland', *Journal of Social Policy*, 35, pp. 97–120.

Kraft, M.E. and Furlong, S.R. (2004) *Public Policy: Politics, Analysis and Alternatives*, Washington, DC: CQ Press.

Krieger, N., Northridge, M., Gruskin, S., Quinn, M., Kriebel, D., Davey-Smith, G., Bassett, M., Rehkopf, D.H. and Millar, C. (2003) 'Assessing health impact assessment: multidisciplinary and international perspectives', *Journal of Epidemiology and Community Health*, 57, pp. 659–62.

Krnv, L. and Thissen, W.A.H. (2000) 'Rationality in decision and policy making: implications for strategic environmental assessment', *Impact Assessment and Project Appraisal*, 18 (3), pp. 191–200.

Landry, C. (2008) *The Creative City: A Toolkit for Urban Innovators*, 2nd edn, London: Earthscan.

Lasswell, H. (1935) *Politics: Who Gets What, When, How*, London: McGraw-Hill.

Lasswell, H.D. (1959) 'Strategies of enquiry: the rational use of observation', in Lerner, D. (ed.) *The Human Meaning of the Social Sciences*, New York: Meridian Books.

Lavin, T. and Metcalfe, O. (2007a) 'Traffic and transport at the local level: capacity building for HIA at the local level in Ireland', in Wismar, M., Blau, J., Ernst, K. and Figueras, J. (eds) *The Effectiveness of Health Impact Assessment: Scope and Limitations of Supporting Decision-Making in Europe*, Copenhagen: WHO Regional Office for Europe.

Lavin, T. and Metcalfe, O. (2007b) 'A city council's air quality action plan: building capacity for HIA in Northern Ireland', in Wismar, M., Blau, J., Ernst, K. and Figueras, J. (eds) *The Effectiveness of Health Impact Assessment: Scope and Limitations of Supporting Decision-Making in Europe*, Copenhagen: WHO Regional Office for Europe.

Lavin, T., Higgins, C., Metcalfe, O. and Jordan, A. (2006) *Health Impacts of the Built Environment: A Review*, Dublin and Belfast: Institute of Public Health.

Leppo, K., Ollila, E., Pena, S., Wismar, M. and Cook, S. (eds) (2013) *Health in All Policies, Seizing Opportunities, Implementing Policies*, Finland: Ministry of Social Affairs and Health, Department for Promotion of Welfare and Health.

Lindblom, C.E. and Woodhouse, E.J. (1993) *The Policy-Making Process*, 3rd edn, New Jersey: Prentice-Hall.

Lindsay, S. (2006) *Health in Our Hands, A Celebration of Achievement: Summary of Ex-Post Evaluation 2001 to 2006 of the Bogside and Brandywell Health Forum*, Derry: Bogside and Brandywell Health Forum.

Littig, B. (2006a) 'Qualitative versus quantitative research methods', Plenary 2, European Consortium for Political Research (ECPR) *Summer School in Research Methods and Techniques*, University of Ljubljana, Slovenija, 7 August.

Lock, K. and McKee, M. (2005) 'Health impact assessment: assessing opportunities and barriers to intersectoral health improvement in an expanded European Union', *Journal of Epidemiology and Community Health*, 59, pp. 356–60.

Lock, K., Gabrijelcic-Blemkus, M., Martuzzi, M., Otorepec, P., Wallace, P., Dora, C., Robertson, A. and Zakotnic, J.M. (2003) 'Health Impact Assessment of agriculture and food policies: lessons learnt from the Republic of Slovenija', *Bulletin World Health Organisation*, 81 (6), pp. 391–8.

Lowndes, V. (2002) 'Institutionalism', in Marsh, D. and Stoker, G. (eds) *Theory and Methods in Political Science*, Hampshire and New York: Palgrave Macmillan.

Lukes, S. (1974) *Power: A Radical View*, London: Macmillan.

Lyons, S. (2005) *Regulatory Impact Assessment in a Small Regional Economy: Applying the New Irish Model.* Lecture presented as for The Policy Institute, Trinity College Dublin, 25 October.

Macrory Report (1970), *Review of Local Government in Northern Ireland* (Cmd 546), Belfast: HMSO.

Mahoney, M. (2009) 'Imperatives for policy health impact assessment: perspectives, positions, power relations'. Unpublished PhD thesis, Deakin University.

Majone, G. (1989) *Evidence, Argument, and Persuasion in the Policy Process*, New Haven: Yale University Press.

March, J.G. and Olsen, J.P. (1984) 'The new institutionalism: organizational factors in political life', *American Journal of Political Science Review*, 78, pp. 734–49.

March, J.G. and Olsen, J.P. (1989) *Rediscovering Institutions: The Organisational Basis of Politics*, New York, London, Toronto, Sydney and Singapore: The Free Press.

March, J.G. and Olsen, J.P. (1995) *Democratic Governance*, New York: Free Press.

March, J.G. and Olsen, J.P. (1996) 'Institutional perspectives on political institutions', *Governance*, 9, pp. 247–64.

March, J.G. and Olsen, J.P. (2005) *Evaluating the 'New Institutionalism'*, Working Paper No. 11, Arena, Centre for European Studies, University of Oslo.

Marmot, M. and Wilkinson, R. (1999) *Social Determinants of Health*, Oxford: Oxford University Press.

Marmot, M.G., Davey Smith, G. and Stansfield, S. (1991) 'Health inequalities among British civil servants: the Whitehall II study', *Lancet*, 337, pp. 1387–93.

Marmot Review Team (2010) *Fair Society, Healthy Lives: A Strategic Review of Health Inequalities in England post-2010*, England: The Marmot Review.

McAuliffe, E. and McKenzie, K. (2007) 'Thinking and acting in healthcare', in E. McAuliffe and K. McKenzie (eds) *The Politics of Healthcare: Achieving Real Reform*, Dublin: The Liffey Press.

McAvoy, H. (2007) *All-Ireland Policy Paper on Fuel Poverty and Health*, Dublin: Institute of Public Health in Ireland.

McKay, C.J. (1991) 'Local government finance in Northern Ireland: why no reform?', *Municipal Journal*.

McKevitt, D. (1990) *Health Care Policy in Ireland: A Study in Control*, Cork: Hibernian University Press.

McSheffrey, G. (2000) *Planning Derry: Planning and Politics in Northern Ireland*, Liverpool: Liverpool University Press.

Metcalfe, O. and Higgins, C. (2009) 'Healthy public policy – is health impact assessment the cornerstone?', *Public Health*, 123, pp. 296–301.

Metcalfe, O., Higgins, C. and Lavin, T. (2009) *Health Impact Assessment Guidance*, Dublin and Belfast: Institute of Public Health in Ireland.

Milio, N. (1981) *Promoting Health through Public Policy*, Philadelphia: FA Davis.

Milio, N. (1990) 'Healthy cities: the new public health and supportive research', *Health Promotion International*, 5, pp. 291–7.

Milliken, M.F. (1959) 'Inquiry and policy: the relation of knowledge into action', in Lerner, D. (ed.) *The Human Meaning of the Social Sciences*, New York: Meridian Books.

Milner, S.J., Bailey, C. and Deans, J. (2003) 'Fit for purpose Health Impact Assessment: a realistic way forward', *Public Health*, 117 (5), pp. 295–300.

Mindell, J., Ison, E. and Joffe, M. (2003) 'A glossary for health impact assessment', *Journal of Epidemiology and Community Health*, 57, pp. 647–51.

Mindell, J.S., Boltong, A. and Forde, I. (2008) 'A review of health impact assessment frameworks', *Public Health*, 122, pp. 1177–87.

Mindell, J., Hansell, A., Morrison, D., Douglas, M. and Joffe, M. (2001) 'What do we need for robust, quantitative Health Impact Assessment?', *Journal of Public Health Medicine*, 23 (3), pp. 173–8.

Mintz, A., Geva, N., Redd, S.B. and Carnes, A. (1997) 'The effect of dynamic and static choice sets on political decision-making: an analysis using the decision board platform', *American Political Science Review*, 91 (3), pp. 533–66.

Mittelmark, M.B. (2000) 'Promoting social responsibility for health: health impact assessment and healthy public policy at the community level', Geneva: WHO.

Mittelmark, M., Gillis, D. and Hsu-Hage, B. (2007) 'Community developement: the role of HIA', in Kemm, J., Parry, J. and Palmer, S. (eds) *Health Impact Assessment: Concepts, Theory, Techniques and Application*, Oxford: Oxford University Press.

Molnar, A., Adam, B., Antova, T., Bosak, L., Dimitrov, P., Pekarcikova, J., Zurlyte, I., Gulis, G., Adany, R. and Kosa, K. (2012) 'Health impact assessment of Roma housing policies in Central and Eastern Europe: a comparative analysis', *Environmental Impact Assessment Review*, 33 (1), pp. 7–14.

Morgan, A. (2006) 'Determinants of health', in Davies, M. and MacDowell, W. (eds) *Health Promotion Theory*, Berkshire: Open University Press.

Morgan, G. (2009) 'On the limitations of health impact assessment', *Public Health*, 123 (12), p. 820.

Morgan, R.K. (2008) 'Institutionalising HIA: the New Zealand experience', *Impact Assessment and Project Appraisal*, 26 (1), pp. 2–16.

Morley, R.L. (2010) 'Systematic review of Housing Interventions and Health: Introduction, Methods, and Summary Findings', *Journal of Public Health Management & Practice*, 16 (5), pp. S5–S10.

Murray, P. (2006) 'The evolution of Irish health policy: a sociological analysis', in McCluskey, D. (ed.) *Health Policy and Practice in Ireland*, Dublin: University College Dublin.

(NCHPP) National Centre for Healthy Public Policy (2011) *Citizen Participation in HIA: An Overview of the Principal Arguments Supporting it*, Fact Sheet, November edition.

Northern Ireland Executive (2001) *Programme for Government*, Belfast: Office of the Minister and Deputy First Minister.

Northern Ireland Executive (2002) *Draft Programme for Government*, Belfast: Office of the First Minister and Deputy First Minister.

Northern Ireland Office (2006) *Better Government for Northern Ireland: Final Decisions of the Review of Public Administration*, Belfast: Northern Ireland Office.

Northern Ireland Statistics and Research Agency (NISRA) (2005) *Northern Ireland Annual Abstract of Statistics*, Belfast: HMSO.

Northern Ireland Statistics and Research Agency (2014a) *Population Clock Northern Ireland*, Belfast: NISRA, available at: www.nisra.gov.uk/population_clock/ClockText.html, accessed 17 February 2014.

Northern Ireland Statistics and Research Agency (2014b) *Interim Life Tables, Northern Ireland (period 2010–2012)*, Belfast: NISRA, available at: www.nisra.gov.uk/demography/default.asp130.htm, accessed 18 February 2014.

OECD (2008) *OECD Public Management Reviews – Ireland: Towards an Integrated Public Service*, Paris: OECD, available at: www.oecd.org/ireland/oecdpublicmanagementreviews-irelandtowardsanintegratedpublicservice.htm#3, accessed 11 February 2014.

O'Faircheallaigh, C. (2010) 'Public participation and EIA: purposes, implications and lessons for public policy', *EIA Review*, 30, pp. 19–27.

Office of First Minister and Deputy First Minister (2005) The Policy Toolkit, available at: www.ofmdfmni.gov.uk/policy-toolkit, accessed 5 February 2014.

O'Mullane, M. (2008) 'Impact assessment in policy-making circles: a lot done, more to do', *PolicyLink*, publication series of the Office of First Minister and Deputy First Minister (OFMDFM), Castle Buildings, Stormont, Belfast.

O'Mullane, M. (2009a) 'The case for health impact assessment in Irish public policy', *Administration*, 56 (4), pp. 87–109.

O'Mullane, M. (2009b) 'An investigation of the utilisation of health impact assessments (HIAs) in Irish public policy making', PhD thesis, University College Cork. Available at: http://cora.ucc.ie/handle/10468/798, accessed 6 February 2014.

O'Mullane, M. (2013) *Integrating Health Impact Assessment with the Policy Process: Lessons and Experiences from around the World*, Oxford: Oxford University Press.

O'Mullane, M. (2014) 'Implementing the legal provisions for Health Impact Assessment in Slovakia: an exploration of practitioner perspectives', *Health Policy* (accepted; forthcoming)

O'Mullane, M. and Guliš, G. (2014) 'Health impact assessment', in Fehr, R., Viliani, F., Nowacki, J. and Martuzzi, M. (eds) *Health in Impact Assessments: Opportunities not to be missed*, Copenhagen: WHO Regional Office for Europe.

O'Mullane, M. and Quinlivan, A. (2012) 'Health impact assessment (HIA) in Ireland and the role of local government', *EIA Review*, 32 (1), pp. 181–6.

O'Neill, C., McGregor, P. and Merkur, S. (2012) 'United Kingdom (Northern Ireland): health system review', *Health Systems in Transition*, 14 (10), pp. 1–91.

O Riain, G. (2005) *From Dogma to Dialogue: Report on the Operation of Local Traveller Accommodation Consultative Committees in County Donegal, Galway City and County Longford*, Donegal: Donegal Travellers Project.

Parry, J. and Scully, E. (2003) 'Health impact assessment and the consideration of health inequalities', *Journal of Public Health*, 25, pp. 243–45.

Parry, J. and Wright, J. (2003) 'Community participation in health impact assessments: intuitively appealing but practically difficult', *Bulletin of the WHO*, 55, pp. 219–20.

Parsons, W. (1995) *Public Policy: An Introduction to the Theory and Practice of Policy Analysis*, Cheltenham and Lyme: Edward Elgar.

Patton, C.V. and Sawicki, D.S. (1993) *Basic Methods of Policy Analysis and Planning*, New Jersey: Prentice Hall.

Patton, M.Q. (1997) *Utilisation-Focused Evaluation*, 3rd edn, Thousand Oaks: Sage Publications.

Peters, B.G. (1999) *Institutional Theory in Political Science: The New Institutionalism*, London and New York: Pinter.

Pobal (2014) RAPID FAQ, available at: www.pobal.ie/FAQ/Pages/RAPID.aspx, accessed 25 February 2014.

Powell, F. (2007) *The Politics of Civil Society: Neoliberalism or Social Left?* Bristol: The Policy Press.

Pursell, L. and Kearns, N. (2012) 'Impacts of an HIA on inter-agency and inter-sectoral partnerships and community participation: lessons from a local level HIA in the Republic of Ireland', *Health Promotion International*, 28 (4), pp. 522–32.

Putters, K. (1996) *Health Impact Screening: Rational Models in their Administrative Context*, Rotterdam: Erasmus University.

Putters, K. (2005) 'Health impact assessment, the next step: defining models and roles', *Environmental Impact Assessment Review*, 25, pp. 693–701.

Quigley, R.J. and Taylor, L.C. (2003) 'Evaluation as a key part of health impact assessment: the English experience', *Bulletin of the World Health Organisation*, 81 (3), pp. 415–19.

Quigley, R., den Broeder, L. Furu, P., Bond, A., Cave, B. and Bos, R. (2006) *Health Impact Assessment International Best Practice Principles. Special Publication Series No. 5*, Fargo, USA: IAIA.

Quin, S. (1999) 'Improving healthy care: health policy in Ireland', in Quin, S., Kennedy, P., O'Donnell, A. and Kiely, G. (eds) *Contemporary Irish Social Policy*, Dublin: University College Dublin Press.

Quinlivan, A. (2013a) Public Community Lecture in Macroom, County Cork, November 2013.

Quinlivan, A. (2013b) 'Councils are vital to the good health of democracy', *Cork Evening Echo*, 25 October 2013.

Quinlivan, A. (2013c) 'Local government reform – real or imaginary', lecture delivered at the spring seminar of the Association of Municipal Authorities of Ireland, New Ross, Wexford, February 2013.

Quinlivan, A. and Cabrol, Y (2013) 'Austerity plans could see Ireland scrap 83 councils – but will it help?', *Guardian*, available at: www.theguardian.com/local-government-network/2013/oct/21/ireland-future-local-government-austerity-reform, accessed 21 October 2013.

Quinlivan, A. (2014) Personal correspondence, 12 February 2014.

Quinlivan, A. and Schön-Quinlivan, E. (2009) 'Innovation and best practice in Irish local government', SIPTU/Chambers Ireland, Dublin.

Quinn, B. (2007) 'People, policies and participation in Irish local government', paper presented the CINEFOGO (Citizen Participation in Policy Making) Conference, Bristol (February).

Rhodes, R.A.W. (1996) 'The institutional approach', in Marsh, D. and Stoker, G. (eds) *Theory and Methods in Political Science*, Basingstoke: Macmillan.

Ritchie, J. and Lewis, J. (2003) *Qualitative Research Practice: A Guide for Social Science Students and Researchers*, Thousand Oaks: Sage Publications.

Rokeach, M. (1973) *Understanding Human Values: Individual and Societal*, New York: The Free Press.

Rossi, P.H., Lipsey, M.W. and Freeman, H.E. (2004) *Evaluation: A Systematic Approach*, 7th edn, Thousand Oaks: Sage Publications.

Sabatier, P.A. (1999) *Theories of the Policy Process*, United States: Westview Press.

Sabatier, P.A. and Jenkins-Smith, H.C. (1993) *Policy Change and Learning: An Advocacy Coalition Approach*, Columbus: Westview Press.

Sanderson, I. (2002) 'Evaluation, policy learning and evidence-based policy-making', *Public Administration*, 80 (1), pp. 1–22.

Saracci, R. (1997) 'The World Health Organisation needs to reconsider its definition of health', *BMJ*, 314, p. 1409.

Scott, P. (2006) 'Development of environmental impact assessment and strategic environmental assessment in Ireland', presentation at the International Association for Impact Assessment UK-Ireland Launch Meeting. *Up, Down and Sideways: Extending and Integrating Assessments*, 24 March. Dublin: UCD.

Scott-Samuel, A. (1996) 'Health impact assessment: an idea whose time has come', *BMJ*, 313, pp. 183–4.

Scott-Samuel, A. (2006) 'Forum chair: healthy public policy', *7th International Health Impact Assessment Conference*, Cardiff, Wales, 5–6 April.

Scott-Samuel, A., Birley, M. and Ardern, K. (1998) *The Merseyside Guidelines for Health Impact Assessment*, Liverpool: The Merseyside Health Impact Assessment Steering Group.

Scott-Samuel, A., Birley, M. and Ardern, K. (2001) *The Merseyside Guidelines for Health Impact Assessment*, 2nd edn, May 2001. Published by the International Health Impact Assessment Consortium.

Silke, D. (2005) 'Accommodating the traveller community', in Norris, M. and Redmond, D. (eds) *Housing in Contemporary Ireland: Policy, Society and Shelter*, Dublin: Institute of Public Administration.

Stake, R.E. (1995) *The Art of Case Study Research*, London and New York: Sage Publications.

Steinberger, P.J. (1993) *The Concept of Political Judgement*, Chicago and London: University of Chicago Press.

Stone, D. (2002) *Policy Paradox: The Art of Political Decision Making*, New York: W.W. Norton.

Taylor, M.S., Wheeler, B.W., White, M.P., Economou, T. and Osborne, N.J. (2015). 'Research note: Urban street tree density and antidepressant prescription rates: A cross-sectional study in London, UK', *Landscape and Urban Planning*, 136, pp. 174–79.

Thelen, K. and Steinmo, S. (1992) 'Historical institutionalism in comparative politics', in Steinmo, S., Thelen, K. and Longstreth, F. (eds) *Structuring Politics: Historical Institutionalism in Comparative Analysis*, Cambridge: Cambridge University Press.

Thomson, H., Kearns, A. and Petticrew, M. (2003) 'Assessing the health impact of local amenities: a qualitative study of contrasting experiences of local swimming pool and leisure provision in two areas of Glasgow', *J Epidemiol Community Health*, 57, pp. 663–7.

Thomson, H., Thomas, S., Sellstrom, E. and Petticrew, M. (2013) 'Housing improvements for health and associated socio-economic outcomes', *Cochrane Database of Systematic Reviews*, 2.

Toland, S. (2006) 'Forward by the environmental health manager', in Ison, E., *Health Impact Assessment of the Draft Air Quality Action Plan for Belfast* (abridged version), Belfast: Belfast City Council (May).

Tonge, J. (2005) *The New Northern Irish Politics?*, Hampshire and New York: Palgrave Macmillan.

Tsouros, A (1990) *World Health Organisation Healthy Cities Project: A Project Becomes a Movement – Review of Progress 1987 to 1990*, Copenhagen, FADL and Milan: Sogess.

Tussing, A.D. and Wren, M.A. (2006) *How Ireland Cares: The Case for Health Care Reform*, Dublin: New Island Press.

UK Healthy Cities Network (2014) *Phase VI* (Healthy Cities), available at: www.healthycities.org.uk/phase-vi-themes.php?s=196, accessed 22 January 2014.

UNECE (2003) 'Protocol on Strategic Environmental Assessment to the Convention on Environmental Impact Assessment in a Transboundary Context, Kiev', available at: www.unece.org/fileadmin/DAM/env/eia/documents/legaltexts/protocolenglish.pdf, accessed 5 February 2014.

URBAN (2002) *HIA for Ballyfermot: Draft Project Proposal Form, Ballyfermot*, Dublin: URBAN II Programme.

Vohra, S., Cave, B., Viliani, F., Harris-Roxas, B. and Bhatia, R. (2010) 'New international consensus on health impact assessment', *The Lancet*, 376, p. 1464.

Voss, J.F. (1998) 'On the representation of problems: an information-processing approach to foreign policy decision making', in Sylvan, D.A. and Voss, J.F. (eds) *Problem Representation in Foreign Policy Decision Making*, Cambridge: Cambridge University Press, pp. 8–26.

Walt, G. (1994) *Health Policy: An Introduction to Process and Power*, London: Zed Books.

Webb, D. (2014) *Public Expenditure by Country and Region*, House of Commons Library, Economic Policy and Statistics Section, London: House of Commons, Westminster.

Weeks, L. and Quinlivan, A. (2009) *All Politics is Local: A Guide to Local Elections in Ireland*, Cork: The Collins Press.

Weimer, D.L. and Vining, A.R. (1992) *Policy Analysis: Concepts and Practice*, 2nd edn, New Jersey: Prentice Hall.

Weimer, D.L. and Vining, A.R. (1999) *Policy Analysis: Concepts and Practice*, 3rd edn, New Jersey: Prentice Hall.

Weiss, C.H. (1977) *Using Social Research in Public Policy-Making*, Toronto: Lexington Books.

Weiss, C.H. (1980) 'Knowledge creep and decision accretion', *Knowledge: Creation, Diffusion, Utilisation*, 1 (3), pp. 381–404.

Weiss, C.H. (1991) 'Policy research: data, ideas or arguments?', in Wagner, P., Weiss, C.H., Wittrock, B. and Wollman, H. (eds) *Social Sciences and Modern States: National Experiences and Theoretical Crossroads*, Cambridge: Cambridge University Press.

Weston, J. (2002) 'From Poole to Fulham: a changing culture in UK environmental impact assessment decision making', *Journal of Environmental Planning and Management*, 45 (3), pp. 425–43.

Wildavsky, A. B. (1979) *Speaking Truth to Power: The Art and Craft of Policy Analysis*, Boston: Little Brown.

Wilford, R., Wilson, R. and Claussen, K. (2007) *Power to the People? Assessing Democracy in Northern Ireland: A TASC Report*, Dublin: Think Tank for Action on Social Change (TASC).

Wilkinson, R. and Marmot, M. (2003) *Social Determinants of Health: The Solid Facts*, 2nd edn, Copenhagen: WHO Regional Office for Europe.

Winkler, M.S., Krieger, G.R., Divall, M.J., Cisse, G., Wielga, M., Singer, B.H., Tanner, M. and Utzinger, J. (2013) 'Untapped potential of health impact assessment', *Bulletin of the World Health Organization*, 91, pp. 298–305.

Wise, M., Harris, P., Harris-Roxas, B. and Harris, E. (2009) 'The role of Health Impact Assessment in promoting population health and health equity', *Health Promotion Journal of Australia*, 20, pp. 172–9.

Wismar, M., Blau, J., Ernst, K. and Figueras, J. (2007) *The Effectiveness of Health Impact Assessment: Scope and Limitations of Supporting Decision-Making in Europe*, Copenhagen: WHO Regional Office for Europe.

Wismar, M., Lahtinen, E., Ståhl, T., Ollila, E. and Leppo, K. (2006) 'Introduction', in Ståhl, T., Wismar, M., Ollila, E., Lahtinen, K. and Leppo, K., *Health in All Policies- Prospects and Potentials*, Ministry of Social Affairs and Health, Finland and European Health Observatory on Health Systems and Policy.

World Health Organization (1946) *Constitution of the World Health Organisation*, Geneva: WHO.

World Health Organization (1978) *Declaration of Alma-Ata International Conference on Primary Health Care*, Alma-Ata, USSR, WHO.

World Health Organization (1979) *Formulating Strategies for Health for All by the Year 2000*, Geneva: WHO.

World Health Organization (1981) *Global Strategy for Health for All by the Year 2000*, Geneva: WHO.

World Health Organization (1986) *Ottawa Charter for Health Promotion*, Geneva: WHO.

World Health Organization (1988) Second International Conference on Health Promotion. Adelaide Recommendations on Healthy Public Policy. Available at: www.who.int/hpr/archive/docs/adelaide, accessed 12 March 2014.

World Health Organization (2013a) *Health 2020: A European Policy Framework and Strategy for the 21st Century*, Copenhagen: WHO Regional Office for Europe.

World Health Organisation (2013b) *Phase VI (2014–2018) of the WHO European Healthy Cities Network: Goals and Requirements*, Copenhagen: WHO Regional Office for Europe.

World Health Organisation (2014) *Phase V- Healthy Cities*, available at: www.euro.who.int/en/health-topics/environment-and-health/urban-health/activities/healthy-cities/who-european-healthy-cities-network/phases-iv-of-the-who-european-healthy-cities-network/phase-v, accessed 22 January 2014.

World Health Organization and United National Environmental Programme (2004) *Health and Environment: Tools for Effective Decision-Making- WHO and UNEP Health and Environment Linkage (HELI)*, Geneva: WHO.

World Health Organization European Centre for Health Policy (1999) *Health Impact Assessment: Main Concepts and Suggested Approach* (Gothenburg Consensus Paper), Brussels: WHO.

Wren, M.A. (2003) *Unhealthy State: Anatomy of a Sick Society*, Dublin: New Island.

Yin, R.K. (2003) *Case Study Research: Design and Methods*, 3rd edn, Thousand Oaks: Sage Publications.

Index